Applications for Medical Practice Success

Kathryn P. Glass, MBA, MSHA

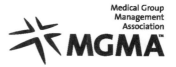

Medical Group
Management
Association

Medical Group Management Association
104 Inverness Terrace East
Englewood, CO 80112
877.275.6462
Web site: www.mgma.com

KENDALL/HUNT PUBLISHING COMPANY
4050 Westmark Drive   Dubuque, Iowa 52002

Cover photo courtesy of PhotoDisc

Item # 5915

Copyright © 2003 by the Medical Group Management Association

ISBN 1-56829-177-9

Printed in the United States of America
10   9   8   7   6   5   4   3   2   1

Contents

About the Authors

KATHRYN P. GLASS, MBA, MSHA

Kathryn Glass started her independent contracting business in July 2002 after seven years with the Medical Group Management Association (MGMA) and its Center for Research. Ms. Glass is a nationally recognized speaker and author on all facets of relative value units. She was responsible for several of the MGMA Center for Research's largest research projects related to relative value units, physician profiling, cost analysis, practice improvement and financial performance. Ms. Glass was a coauthor and editor of the *Chart of Accounts for Health Care Organizations,* and is the author of numerous published articles. She was MGMA's subject matter expert on its relative value unit cost accounting distance learning program.

Ms. Glass has master's degrees in business administration and in health care administration from the University of Colorado at Denver.

JEFFREY B. MILBURN, MBA, CMPE

Jeff Milburn is currently the senior vice president for the Colorado Springs Health Partners, P.C., a 65-physician multispecialty practice with nearly 50 percent managed care and 12 locations in Colorado Springs, Colorado. Formerly the chief financial officer, he is currently responsible for managed care contracting and support. Mr. Milburn has more than 20 years of physician practice management and consulting experience.

Group practice managed care, financial management and income distribution plans are areas of particular interest and experience. Milburn has also presented programs and workshops for MGMA and other organizations on a variety of health care finance topics. Mr. Milburn, who has a master's degree in business administration, is board-certified in medical practice management by the American College of Medical Practice Executives (ACMPE). Mr. Milburn had 10 years of commercial banking and finance experience prior to entering the health care management field. He is active in various community activities including the Chamber of Commerce.

ROBERT W. ELLIS, CPA, CMPE

Rob Ellis has more than 15 years of experience in the accounting profession. He has been at Charlotte Orthopedic Specialists (COS) in Charlotte, North Carolina since January 1994 where he was the controller for two years, prior to moving to his current position as the chief financial officer. COS has 40 orthopedic surgeons, 10 physician assistants, 20 therapists and 10 locations. While COS has no capitation contracts, 57 percent of its revenue is generated from managed care.

Mr. Ellis is a nationally renowned speaker and instructor on cost accounting, financial management, cost analysis and RVUs. He earned his business administration degree from the University of North Carolina at Chapel Hill. He is also a certified public accountant and is board-certified in medical practice management by the American College of Medical Practice Executives.

TERRY J. BRENNAN, FACMPE, FHFMA

Terry J. Brennan is a principal in Resource Management Associates, LLC, a management consulting firm specializing in operational functions of health care organizations including strategic planning, managed care contracting, finance and accounting, accounts receivable management, facilities planning, human resources and information services.

Before forming this firm, Mr. Brennan spent a year as vice president of a $57 million health care management services organization. Prior to that position, he served for 15 years as the executive director for the Washington University Department of Surgery, and for seven years as the director of financial management for the Washington School of Medicine.

Mr. Brennan is an active member and a Fellow in the American College of Medical Practice Executives and in the Healthcare Financial Management Association (HFMA). A native of St. Louis, Mr. Brennan holds a master's degree in business administration from Washington University in St. Louis.

JEFF ANDERSON, M.MGT.

Jeff Anderson worked three years as a research associate for the MGMA Center for Research. Prior to that, Jeff accumulated nine years of health care business office experience, including six years in a community health center where he rapidly advanced through the ranks from billing clerk to business manager. Mr. Anderson has written numerous articles on the use of RVUs in practice management. He currently works for the National Association of Community Health Centers.

Mr. Anderson earned his master's degree in health care management from the University of Mary in Bismarck, North Dakota. He received his bachelor's degree in business administration from North Dakota State University in Fargo, North Dakota.

JOHN MENDEZ

Since 1998 John Mendez has been employed by the MGMA Center for Research. Currently a project manager, Mr. Mendez works with various aspects of the RVU-based practice management software tool Physician Services Practice Analysis (PSPA); he participates in the development and testing of the latest version of the software and assists in the production of the PSPA comparison report. He is also the primary PSPA technical support contact.

Mr. Mendez has a bachelor's degree in environmental studies from the University of Colorado at Boulder.

Acknowledgments

Heartfelt thanks to Rob Ellis and Jeff Milburn who taught me everything I know about RVU cost accounting, managed care contracting and physician compensation. Special thanks to Len Lichtenfeld who pointed out some of the finer points of RVU expense distribution that I hadn't considered.

I also appreciate the contributions of Brian Roth from the University of Iowa Community Medical Services and Terry Brennan of Resource Management Consultants. Their real-life examples of physician compensation packages made that chapter much more tangible to the readers. A lot of thought and effort goes into compensation packages. I sincerely appreciate their willingness to share their experiences with us.

Finally, I wish to acknowledge and thank reviewers Len Lichtenfeld, Beth Lindroos and Leanne Travers for their time, effort and detailed comments. Having a fresh set of eyes on the authors' work really helped to clarify and expand on ideas presented.

Kathryn Glass

CHAPTER **1**

Introduction to RVUs

INTRODUCTION

Knowledge is power. It's not just having data, but having the knowledge born of a thorough data analysis that leads to the power. Medical groups have tons of clinical data, but they typically lack a method of common-denominator analyses and per-unit comparisons for all the clinical productivity and expense data. That type of analysis would provide the practice administrators with the knowledge—and therefore the power—to make proactive and informed decisions. Although originally developed and implemented through several different scales over the last few decades as an equitable payment mechanism for physician services, relative value units (RVUs) have evolved far beyond that initial intention. Exactly what are RVUs? Where did they come from? How do they differ from encounters and fees in terms of measuring provider productivity? How can they be used to increase cost effectiveness and maximize productivity within medical practices? The answers to those questions and more are included within this book. Ideally, however, actual RVU data analysis will raise even more questions, such as why certain providers seem to be more productive and/or more cost effective than their peers. While those are questions that the authors of this book cannot answer directly, we can show you ways of uncovering the truth. RVU data analysis provides the quantitative power that comes with this knowledge.

WHAT ARE RVUS?

RVUs are nonmonetary, relative units of measure that indicate the value of health care services and relative differences in resources consumed when providing different procedures and services. Simply stated, RVUs are supposed to be an objective, standardized method of analyzing resources involved in the provision of services or procedures. RVUs assign *relative* values or weights to medical procedures primarily for the purpose of reimbursement of services performed and secondarily for internal productivity measurements and cost analysis, although that was not their original purpose. RVUs are also used in external benchmarking against better performing practices, although exactly what constitutes the best practices is still being defined within the medical community.

It is equally important to realize the limitations of RVUs. RVUs are *not* risk adjusters, case severity adjusters, determinants of coding compliance or medical diagnostic tools. This is a critical distinction that needs to be made in order to understand what RVUs can and cannot provide in terms of practice management tools.

HISTORY OF RVUS

RVUs are assigned to medical common procedural terminology (CPT) codes copyrighted by the American Medical Association (AMA) and to the current dental terminology (CDT) codes copyrighted by the American Dental Association (ADA). CPTs and CDTs each have their own RVU systems built on different scales. Anesthesia services (CPT code range 00100 – 01999) also has its own relative value scale developed by the American Society of Anesthesiologists (ASA) and subsequently adopted by the Health Care Financing Administration (HCFA) as the methodology for reimbursing anesthesiology services under the Medicare program. The Centers for Medicare and Medicaid Services' (CMS, formerly HCFA) Resource-Based Relative Value Scale (RBRVS) is the current industry standard for benchmarking, provider compensation, third-party payer reimbursement and health services cost analysis. It is the system most widely used for medical procedures; however, it is not the only RVU system in existence.

CMS's RBRVS

A Harvard University School of Public Health research team head-
ed by Dr. William C. Hsiao, and funded by what was then HCFA, originally developed the methodology behind the CMS's RBRVS. The system was developed to recognize objective measures of physician work
and to provide a more acceptable and perhaps more competitive payment system for physicians across all specialties providing care to
Medicare beneficiaries. Prior to the development of the RBRVS, the
universally accepted method of reimbursement was based upon customary, prevailing and reasonable (CPR) charges.[1] Until the advent of
the RBRVS, even the existing relative value scales were based upon
physicians' charges, which simply perpetuated the market's price dis-
tortions.[2,3] Because of the variation in charges and payments due, in
large part, to the geographic variability and the fiscal constraints
imposed by Medicare in the mid-1970s and early 1980s, dissatisfac-
tion with the CPR system increased for some physicians. For others,
such as surgeons, the CPR system was quite satisfactory because surgeries were high-revenue producers and quite profitable in many
cases.

Requests to change and improve the system of reimbursement
began with physicians, the AMA, insurance companies and the government; however, this change began predominantly with primary
care organizations that were faced with an increasing shortfall in revenues under CPR. It was clear that with CPR there was little equiva-
lence between evaluation/management services and surgical services.
Consequently, CMS contracted with the Harvard group to develop the
RBRVS, which, since its implementation in January 1992, has evolved
into an industry standard for physician reimbursement. The methodology used in the development of the RBRVS included calculating the
effort of providing each procedure in each of three areas: physician
work, practice expense (overhead) and malpractice. Dr. Hsiao's work
focused on the physician work component.

The development of the RBRVS system took many years and a lot
of cooperative effort from all parties. Technical consulting groups
(TCGs) comprising more than 200 physicians were organized into 33
specialty-specific consulting groups to provide guidance on the study
structure and to define physician work. Vignettes were created to

specifically describe the clinical content of each service so that uniform definitions could be written and clearly understood by all physicians nationwide.[4] The TCGs defined physicians' total work as encompassing both time and intensity.[5] Intensity included mental effort, clinical judgment, technical skill, physical effort and stress related to risk. Total work was divided into three time periods: preservice, intra-service and post-service. In an attempt to provide a readily defensible method of valuing "work effort," the use of magnitude estimation, a means of measuring subjective perceptions and judgments, was employed to measure physicians' subjective perceptions of procedure time and complexity when rating services. The use of magnitude estimation had proved to be reliable and had produced valid results in other previous studies.[6]

The primary objective of the Harvard study was the measurement of the physician work component rather than all three components.[7] In a nutshell, a cross-section of physicians determined the relative amount of work, time and effort that encompassed various procedures they performed. Relative to *what* was the original challenge. The anchor code from which the entire RBRVS was developed was 99213, an established patient office visit with face-to-face time with a physician lasting approximately 15 minutes. At the genesis of the RBRVS the total RVUs assigned to CPT 99213 were 1.0 (it has since changed). The physicians' task was to determine what value should be assigned to other codes relative to 99213 and its value of 1.0. Thus began the process of the RBRVS development. It continues today through a standing committee called the RBRVS Update Committee (RUC) that is dedicated to providing annual updates.

Note that until 2002 not all three RVU components were resource based, even though the scale has always been called the "resource-based relative value scale." It was a bit of a misnomer since only the work component was, in fact, resource based at the beginning. Until the late 1990s the practice expense and the professional liability components were computed by HCFA using a formula that included average Medicare approved charges.[8] The Medicare reimbursement for the practice expense component was calculated by multiplying a percentage of gross revenues that a specialty practice spent on overhead (practice expenses) by the historical payment for a procedure or service.[9] The malpractice component was converted from actual claims-paid data values to resource-based values as of the year 2000. Resource-based practice expense values were phased in over a four-year period completed in 2002. Understandably, this was a source of some confusion and frustration on the part of practice administrators attempting to trend RVU data over the years. With changing values each year, it has been difficult at best to compare one year's productivity and costs to the next using RVUs. Now that the RBRVS is fully resource based, the values should have minimal annual changes. Each of the components is still scheduled for comprehensive five-year reviews, however, so changes over time are inevitable.

CMS's RBRVS comprises the CPT-4 codes, brief descriptions and the RVUs associated with each code. The RBRVS also contains CMS's common procedure coding system (HCPCS), which is a standardized method or system for reporting professional services, procedures and supplies. HCPCSs are typically paid on a flat rate and therefore do not have RVUs assigned to the codes, since none are required to calculate a reimbursement rate. The RBRVS is not copyrighted because its source is a federal government agency, and therefore it is considered public domain. As previously mentioned, the AMA holds the copyright on the CPT-4 codes. This has been a source of some confusion in the past, as people often think of the RBRVS and RVUs as being synonymous, while in reality the RVUs constitute only one part of the entire RBRVS.

Finally, lest the reader think that the RBRVS is the pinnacle of health services measurement, it needs to be pointed out that the current RBRVS has its limitations as well as its strengths. While inputs are carefully measured, the RBRVS does not consider health care outcomes (i.e., output), quality of care or demand for services.[10] RVUs do not take into consideration practice efficiencies or inefficiencies. In addition, not all codes (for example, laboratory and HCPCS) have RVUs assigned, which makes it more difficult, albeit not impossible, to place a standardized value on those procedures and/or services. As Salvador Dali said, "Have no fear of perfection; you'll never reach it." So it is true with RVUs, which continue to evolve with health services.

Relative Values for Physicians

St. Anthony's *Relative Values for Physicians* (RVP) publication (formerly published by McGraw-Hill) provides values both for services that are contained in the Medicare Physicians' Fee Schedule (MPFS) and for procedures and services that are either not yet reimbursable by Medicare or that are reimbursed on a flat-fee basis (for example, laboratory tests). The methodology used to develop the McGraw-Hill scale consisted of a random sample of physicians from across the United States, who were asked to rate specific procedures as to time, skill, risk to the patient, risk to the provider and severity of illness of each.[11] The resulting values were tabulated and resulted in the work component for a given procedure.

These McGraw-Hill relative value units were aligned with Medicare's RBRVS by examining them along with Medicare's work RVU to develop a comparative factor for use between the two systems. The examination process included collecting and listing all codes from each procedure code section that had a McGraw-Hill RVP and a MPFS work value. Values for each group were totaled. The sum of the MPFS work values was divided by the sum of the McGraw-Hill RVP values. This initial comparative factor was then multiplied by the existing McGraw-Hill RVP value for each code. The resulting converted RVP value for each code was then subtracted from the current work values from the MPFS. All codes with differences greater than two standard deviations from the mean were removed from the data sets. The comparative factor was then recalculated using the remaining data. Because the McGraw-Hill RVPs were developed separately, different value scales were used for surgery, radiology, pathology, medicine, and evaluation and management (E&M) sections. The comparative factor from the secondary analysis was then multiplied by the current RVP value for each code, and the product was then used to establish work values for each code for which no value existed in the MPFS. The practice expense and malpractice values for the codes were extracted using percentages determined by CMS for similar procedures.

The system employed by St. Anthony/McGraw-Hill, while introducing a different technical aspect of calculating physician work or effort, is still dependent upon the basic methodology and premise developed by the Harvard group (its original use of CMS percentages to determine practice expense and malpractice) for use in the MPFS. However, at least one physician who is intimately familiar with the development and continual updates behind the RBRVS would argue that the St. Anthony RVP scale is not using anything close to the methodology established by Hsaio et al.

The main differences between the St. Anthony/McGraw-Hill RVP scale and the RBRVS are that the St. Anthony/McGraw-Hill scale

- does not break out the physician work component;
- is a compilation of five independent scales (medicine, surgery, radiology/pathology, laboratory and E&M) instead of one; and
- is focused more on specialty care than primary care.

In addition, the St. Anthony/McGraw Hill scale contains laboratory procedure values not found in the RBRVS. These values cannot and should not be used for comparison purposes with other scales within the RVP or with the RBRVS. The RVUs for laboratory codes are based on their own unique value scale. CMS reimburses for lab procedures on a flat fee; therefore no RVUs are needed for those codes in the RBRVS.

Relative Time-Cost Unit

About the same time that the RBRVS debuted in 1992, a system for the valuation of dental procedures and the development of dental fees based on provider effort was initiated. This system, loosely based on the medical RVU system, is called the Relative Time-Cost Unit (RTCU) system.[12] The dental community faced many of the same issues as the medical community relative to the establishment of fees. Were the fees established reflective of the cost to provide the service? A system that would enable the dental community to move away from tradition and market perception was required. The RTCU system incorporates personnel costs, task mixes and task times into relative weights for valuation of dental procedures. The difference between this and other studies similar in design is that this study utilized more direct task analysis, incorporating actual procedure times and personnel mix to quantify selected dental procedures. In this study a dental assistant's 40-hour salary is indexed at 1.00, a dental hygienist's salary is indexed at 1.83 and a general dentist's salary carries a weight of 4.02. In determining the relative value of a procedure, the relative weights of the personnel performing the service multiplied by the median time required to perform the procedure provide the RTCU.

Although they are referenced here to assist the reader in understanding that differences do exist among the different scales, dental procedures and the corresponding RVUs are outside the scope of this book.

Furthermore, even though there is an RVU scale specifically designed for dental services, the dental community in general claims that the RVU system is irrelevant to the dental environment based on the three following factors:

1. **Medicare does not cover routine dental services.** Unlike medical services, Medicare does not cover routine dental services; therefore, most dental practices are excluded from Medicare's RBRVS reimbursement methodology. As a result, RVUs are not directly linked to dental practice reimbursement. Medicare does, however, cover some oral surgery procedures due to certain illnesses and/or injuries, according to the oral surgeons who are active RUC members.

2. **Commercial third-party dental plans do not utilize RVUs for calculating dental service reimbursement.** Dental commercial payers calculate reimbursement for dental services based on an average charge per procedure minus an adjustment percentage. Again, unlike the medical community where over 50 percent of the third-party payers utilize established physician fee schedules based on a factor of Medicare's physician fee schedule, the dental community's reimbursement does not depend on RVUs.

3. **A national dentist shortage is creating greater demand for dental services.** Most dental practices are operating at maximum capacity, and therefore monitoring dental productivity based on RVUs is not a primary concern for the dental community at this time.

MISCELLANEOUS VALUE METHODOLOGIES

There have been other methodologies addressed in the literature that have attempted to measure and/or assign value to effort and time expended by medical professionals. One such effort involved the study of medical school faculty and attempted to develop an easily modifiable means to ascertain the productivity of medical school faculty in the areas of administration, patient care, teaching and research. In this study, relative values ranging from 1 to 10 were assigned to specific components of each of the four selected areas.[13] The relative values were based upon the level of complexity and time associated with a specified task. For example, in the area of patient care, giving grand rounds was assigned a value of 10, and providing patient care on a half-day basis earned a value of two. A time component was then developed that consisted primarily of estimates of anticipated time required to perform a given activity. The resulting data were then aggregated to arrive at a total that represented the productivity of a particular professor. The development of this study very closely mirrored the development efforts of the RBRVS system, and it serves to further solidify the use of RBRVS as a methodology for the measurement of time and effort for providers of medical services.

Anesthesia Relative Values

RVUs are also assigned to anesthesia codes; however, these values do not follow the methodology used in the RBRVS, and therefore are difficult to compare with medical procedures. Anesthesia services have nothing to do with relative work and everything to do with absolute time. Because of this distinction, anesthesia services cannot be easily converted into anything resembling RBRVS at this time.

According to the American Society of Anesthesiologists,[14] relative value units assigned to anesthesia service CPT codes (00100–01999) are determined by adding a base value (related to case complexity) to the associated time units (typically 10 to 15 minute time blocks), plus applicable modifier units based on particular circumstances of that case, such as patient acuity, if needed. The base value assigned to an anesthesiology CPT code includes the pre- and post-operative visits, plus the typical duties and responsibilities of the physician anesthesiologist in the operating room throughout the surgery.

Mark Meisel, MBA, vice president and chief operating officer for Anesthesia Associates of Kansas City, adds, "Utilizing RVUs as a tool for measuring anesthesiology productivity or costs is difficult because we use both the RBRVS RVU system as well as the ASA's Relative Value Guide (RVG) system depending on what type of service we provide (anesthesia vs. central lines vs. pain management vs. critical care). Additionally, there are practices that use nurse anesthetists and/or residents and some that don't. You could get vastly different production results based on the 'care team' vs. physician-only approach."

Pathology Services

Of the 1,100 pathology and laboratory services defined in the AMA's CPT manual, less than 100 are recognized as physician pathology services under Medicare law and have assigned RVUs within the RBRVS. These services require that doctors of pathology perform these procedures and that pathology service providers must bill Medicare and Medicaid directly for services.

Most of the remaining 1,000-plus services are considered clinical diagnostic laboratory services and are paid based on Medicare's Clinical Laboratory fee schedule which is based on inflation-indexed, reasonable charges rather than RVUs. For these services, it is suggested that medical practices analyze laboratory service utilization, productivity and costs based on procedure frequency, cost per procedure and average reimbursement per procedure.

RVU COMPONENTS

The RBRVS RVUs are divided into three components: the work (officially "physician work") involved in performing a clinical service denoted by RVU_w, the practice expense (RVU_{pe}) associated with delivering the service and the malpractice risk (RVU_m) costs associated with performing the service. Exhibit 1 provides an example of the CPT-4 codes, descriptions, the assigned RVU components and totals (RVU_t). Some RVU purists still use the original verbiage *physician work,* but because that excludes nonphysician providers who bill out for the clinical services they provide using their own unique provider identification code, the terms *provider work* or simply *work* have gained in popularity during recent years.

That is not to say that nonphysician providers receive the same reimbursement from third-party payers that physicians do. In many cases reimbursement is lower for nonphysician providers than for physicians. After all, nonphysician providers do not have the same level of skill, education and scope of services that physicians do, and are, therefore, also compensated at lower levels than those of physicians. Nonphysician providers do, however, bill out for many of the same medical procedures and services that physicians do, and, therefore, may be legitimately included in the discussion of the work component. Some nonphysician providers have a great deal of autonomy, whereas others are viewed more as physician extenders who provide supplemental and/or support work to the physicians. The differences vary by medical practice, by state and by carrier. For example, some states allow dietitians to bill for services they provide, while in other states the bills go out under the physician's name and ID. Whether the service provider is a physician or a nonphysician, the RVUs are not affected unless a modifier is attached to the CPT code.

As seen in Exhibit 1.1, the relative differences among these three codes in resources consumed are evident in the RVUs assigned to each one. A physician's office visit for an established patient where face-to-face time spent with the doctor is approximately 10 minutes vs. obstetrical care (for example, vaginal delivery) is a drastic example of the differences in resources consumed.

Considering resources consumed in the provision of medical procedures and services, exactly what resources are involved? Typically the work expense includes the physicians' and/or nonphysician providers' compensation including benefits. Practice expense includes the entire overhead category, such as staff salaries, supplies, equipment, building expenses, utilities and taxes. Malpractice expense includes the medicolegal risk involved with the provision of each

EXHIBIT 1.1. Examples of RVU Components

CPT-4	Brief Description	RVU_w	RVU_{pe}	RVU_m	RVU_t
99212	Office visit/established patient	0.45	0.59	0.02	1.06
44370	Endoscopy	4.80	1.74	0.21	6.75
59400	Obstetrical care	23.06	15.41	4.14	42.61

service. This is discussed in greater detail when costs per component are covered in chapter 3.

Why should it matter that the total RVUs are split into three separate components? As you begin to work with RVUs in tracking productivity and costs, it will become important to break out the work component from the practice expense (i.e., overhead) and malpractice units. Some clinics, such as those that receive Section 330 grant funding from the federal government, do not have malpractice insurance premiums. Those particular health service clinics are covered by the Federal Tort Claims Act (FTCA), and, therefore, have no need to track this component or to calculate the cost of it in the provision of services. If a practice is developing a provider compensation formula based on RVUs, the practice expense and malpractice RVUs need to be carved out because the compensation should be based strictly on work (clinical productivity) and not on overhead.

In the 2002 RBRVS, the RVU work component accounts for an *average* of approximately 51.4 percent of the total relative value for all procedures (minus those that include technical component [TC] and/or "26 modifiers" to avoid duplication of any procedure). The TC modifier is used for those codes where there is no physician involvement (i.e., work) involved in the service or procedure. The 26 modifier is the professional component. Modifiers are discussed in further detail in chapter 2 on productivity. Practice expense represents an average of 43.1 percent of the total RVUs, and malpractice insurance comprises the remaining 5.5 percent. These proportions vary with each service category, such as surgery, medicine, E&M, etc. For example, using the nonfacility RVUs for E&M CPT codes (99201 to 99499), the work component comprises an average of 62.4 percent, the practice expense 35.2 percent and the malpractice 2.4 percent. As of the 2002 edition of the RBRVS, the relative values are completely resource based for all three components.

Facility and nonfacility RVUs were introduced in the 1998 version of the RBRVS to account for the differences in practice expenses when the medical procedure was performed in a physician's office (i.e., nonfacility) versus another setting. Examples of facility settings include hospitals (inpatient or outpatient), emergency rooms, skilled nursing facilities and ambulatory surgery centers. Nonfacility RVUs are slightly higher because of the direct consumption of the medical practice's resources in the provision of services or procedures. Facility RVUs result in lower reimbursement to the physician than non-facility RVUs because the physician, in a manner of speaking, is not consuming the resources of his or her own office. To clarify the practice expense determination, there is reimbursement for the indirect expenses of the practice, and there are reimbursements for the direct expenses linked to a facility-based procedure. CMS does make an allowance for the expense of maintaining an office while the physician is off in the facility.

Not every code has both facility and nonfacility RVUs assigned because not all services can be performed in all settings. For example, cesarean deliveries and brain surgeries are not normally performed as outpatient procedures in a physician's office, but rather in a hospital setting; therefore, facility RVUs are more appropriate for the practice expense components of those codes. Note that the designation of facility and nonfacility affects only the practice expense component. The work and professional liability components remain unchanged.

CMS's Payment Methodology

Medicare, unlike most insurance carriers that have a variety of conversion factors (CF) for each contract depending in part on geographic location, has only one CF for the entire United States. A conversion factor is simply the number or factor by which RVUs are multiplied in order to calculate a reimbursement for a procedure. A conversion factor converts RVUs into dollars by using a monetary figure. This is explained and examples are given throughout the book. In Exhibit 1.2 the conversion factor is $36.1992. Recognizing that operating costs vary with location, CMS created geographic practice cost indices (GPCIs) to adjust for those differences. For example, it generally costs more to operate a clinic in urban New York City or Los Angeles than it does a similar clinic in rural North Dakota. GPCI adjustments, unique to the Medicare payment system, allow for the variance in expenses so that each practice is equitably reimbursed.

GPCIs have the same three components as the RVUs in the RBRVS, and are typically updated on an annual basis. Both the GPCIs

EXHIBIT 1.2. Reimbursement Calculation Using the Geographic Practice Cost Indices

CPT code 99213: $RVU_w = 0.67$ $RVU_{pe} = 0.69$ $RVU_m = 0.03$

Colorado GPCIs: $GPCI_w = 0.985$ $GPCI_{pe} = 0.992$ $GPCI_m = 0.840$

Medicare's fee schedule calculations:

$[(RVU_w * GPCI_w) + (RVU_{pe} * GPCI_{pe}) + (RVU_m * GPCI_m)] * CF =$ Reimbursement

$[(0.67 * 0.985) + (0.69 * 0.992) + (0.03 * 0.840)] * 36.1992 =$

$(0.65995 + 0.68448 + 0.0252) * 36.1992 =$

$1.36963 * 36.1992 = \$49.58$

and the RBRVS are published by CMS annually in an issue of the *Federal Register* available in early November for the following calendar year. To calculate a Medicare physician's fee schedule, each RVU component for a given CPT code is first multiplied by its corresponding GPCI. The three components are then summed and multiplied by the Medicare CF. The following example shows the reimbursement that a nonfacility (such as an ambulatory care facility) in Colorado would have received from Medicare for office visit code 99213 in the year 2002:

CMS has assigned the state of Colorado GPCI values of less than 1.0, indicating that it is slightly less expensive to operate a practice in Colorado than in some other parts of the U.S., such as Alaska or Rhode Island. Insurance carriers that do not incorporate GPCIs into the fee schedules simply multiply the total RVUs by a conversion factor. Sometimes carriers pay a factor of the RBRVS when reimbursing physicians. For example, a carrier that pays 110 percent of Medicare may calculate the reimbursement for CPT code 99213 with a total RVU of 1.39 (prior to any GPCI adjustment) as follows: 1.39 * 36.1992 * 1.10 = $55.35. If a carrier is competing in Colorado and basing fees on the RBRVS, it may offer less than 100 percent of the RBRVS, since Medicare pays less in Colorado than in some other states. For example, a carrier paying 98 percent of the RBRVS may calculate its fee to match Medicare's payment for 99213 as follows: 1.39 * 36.1992 * 0.98 = $49.31.

More discussion of managed care contracts and various payment methodologies can be found in chapter 4.

Uses of RVUs

As previously noted, the RBRVS was originally designed by CMS for Medicare reimbursement of physician services, but it has since expanded into other uses. CMS is the nation's largest health care purchaser with Medicare/Medicaid coverage for more than 70 million U.S. citizens. As the U.S. population ages (or more to the point as the baby boomer generation ages and becomes eligible for Medicare coverage), this number will continue to rise. According to the American Association of Health Plans' 1998 annual report, more than half (56.3 percent) of the Health Maintenance Organizations (HMOs) paying fee-for-service to primary care physicians and to specialists base their fees on the Medicare fee schedule (i.e., the RBRVS) or a factor of it.[15] The remaining HMOs use either their own fee schedules or other fee schedules that may or may not be modified to meet each HMO's needs. With the majority of health plans using the RBRVS as a payment mechanism, it would serve the practice well to learn to maximize both reimbursements and revenues through RVU cost accounting, RVU productivity analysis, and, finally, through RVU contract negotiation. All of this is done at the per-unit basis—in this case relative unit basis—using the RBRVS.

Provider productivity can be measured in nonfinancial terms through the use of RVUs, since RVUs do not reflect the exact dollar value of any medical procedure to the medical group. The use of RVUs also eliminates any bias included in the practice's charges. Tracking productivity based on RVUs, in addition to or in place of net charges, is now common in provider compensation packages. Other uses for RVUs in productivity measurements include tracking office volume and staffing needs, reviewing composition of top volume codes to determine changes in practice trends and treatment protocols, performing market-based comparisons, monitoring provider performance and providing feedback on improving efficiency and productivity. Although not comprehensive, the list provides food for thought on the potential extent of RVU analyses.

Cost accounting using RVUs as the unit of measurement is a growing trend among medical group practices. Costing of RVUs is discussed in detail in chapter 3. Practice management as a whole can benefit from RVU analysis applied to strategic planning, resource allocation, budgeting, provider compensation, cost-based fee schedules, payer analysis, contract review and maintenance, per procedure profitability, etc. RVU analysis can be used as a tool to increase profitability within a group. Outside the practice, benchmarking tools are available from the Medical Group Management Association (MGMA) and other sources for practices to compare their cost and utilization per RVU and other per unit bases to their peers.

Another use of RVU analysis is in the area of mergers and acquisitions or the sale or purchase of a medical practice. Detailed analysis can be very helpful in determining historical productivity and costs at the group, specialty or provider levels. Looking at trends in these data spanning a period of several years can offer a great deal of insight. (Preferably such analysis should take place *prior* to signing any contracts—a point after which insight turns into hindsight!)

While RVUs offer a greater level of detail in reporting and in productivity and cost analyses than encounters and/or net charges or fees, it is noteworthy to mention that proper coding and compliance are key to accurate analyses and comparisons. If a bias exists in the coding, the bias will also be reflected in the RVUs. This is discussed in chapter 2 on productivity, since it is an integral part of the overall clinical productivity process.

CONCLUSION

While RVUs are not perfect, they do offer more objective, statistically valid measurements of clinical activity and costs than any other methodology currently available. RVUs are an objective, standardized method of analyzing resources involved in the provision of services or procedures. On the other hand, RVUs are *not* risk adjusters, case severity adjusters, determinants of coding compliance or medical diagnostic tools. The RBRVS is the industry's current standard for physician reimbursement, productivity and cost measurements, and benchmarking; therefore, this book focuses on that specific RVU scale.

If this book does not satisfy your thirst for knowledge on RVUs, you may want to check first with MGMA's Information Center or the MGMA Health Care Consulting Group, an excellent source for the latest information on RVUs and their uses. In addition, the *Journal of Medical Practice Management* has published a series of four articles on RVUs written by this author and published in 2002. Other resources include past issues of *Healthcare Financial Management* magazine from the Healthcare Financial Management Association and the *Physician Compensation Report* published by Atlantic Information Services, Inc. (AIS).

Notes

1. American Medical Association. (2000, January). Medicare RBRVS: The Physicians' Guide, Chicago, 4–33.
2. California Medical Association. (1969). 1969 Relative Value Studies. San Francisco.
3. Hadley, J., Juba, D., Berenson, RD., Swartz, K., Wagener, J. (1984). Final Report on Alternative Methods of Developing a Relative Value Scale of Physicians' Services. Washington, DC: The Urban Institute.
4. Verrilli, DK., Dunn, DL., Sulvetta, MB. (1996, October). The Measurement of Physician Work and Alternative Uses of the Resource Based Relative Value Scale. Journal of Ambulatory Care Management 19(4):40, 42–48.
5. Hsiao, WC., Braun, P., Dunn, D., Becker, ER., Yntema, D., Verrilli, DK, Stamenovic, E., Chen, S. (1992, November). An Overview of the Development and Refinement of the Resource-Based Relative Value Scale, Medical Care, 30(11) Supplement.
6. Bohrnstedt, GW. (1969). A Quick Method for Determining the Reliability and Validity of Multiple-Item Scales, AM Social Rev 34:542.
7. Verrilli, DK., Dunn, DL., Sulvetta, MB. (1996, October). The Measurement of Physician Work and Alternative Uses of the Resource Based Relative Value Scale. Journal of Ambulatory Care Management 19(4):40, 42–48.
8. American Medical Association. (1997). RVS Update Process. Chicago.
9. Lichtenfeld, JL. (1995). The RBRVS: Fixing the Flaws. The Internist: Health Policy in Practice. 36(9): 13–16.
10. Becker, ER., Dunn, D., Braun, P., Hsiao, WC. (1990). Refinement and Expansion of the Harvard Resource-Based Relative Value Scale: The Second Phase. American Journal of Public Health 80(7): 799–803.
11. Relative Value Studies, Inc. (1995). The McGraw-Hill Complete RBRVS.
12. Marcus, M., Koch, AL., Schoen, MH., Tuominen, R. (1990, October). A proposed New System for Valuing Dental Procedures—The Relative Time—Cost Unit. Medical Care, 28(10).

13. Hilton, C., Fisher, W., Jr., Lopez, A., Sanders, C. (1997, September). A Relative Value Based System for Calculating Faculty Productivity in Teaching, Research, Administration, and Patient Care, Academic Medicine, 72(9).
14. American Society of Anesthesiologists. Relative Value Guide. (1992).
15. Fitzgerald, P., Maples, CT. (1998). AAHP Annual Industry Survey, 1998. 1999 Industry Profile: A Health Plan Reference Book. 96.

CHAPTER 2

Productivity as Measured by RVUs

INTRODUCTION

Traditionally, medical groups tracked a provider's clinical productivity based in part on the following: total gross charges; total net medical revenue or total cost; patient panel size; growth rate of patient base; hospital admissions, visits or consults; office hours, practice coverage, procedural volume or number of cases; and/or RVU production. This list is by no means exhaustive, but it does indicate that no one measure of productivity was used in the past, nor should just one measure be used now. It is important to note that RVUs measure only clinical activity—not administrative, teaching or research activities. This is a primary reason why RVUs should not be the *only* measure of activity within any medical practice, especially if the physicians are involved in administration, teaching and research, as they would be in an academic setting. Productivity as discussed in this text is limited to clinical activity that can be measured by RVUs.

Frequently, medical practices base the majority of their clinical productivity measures on encounters, fees or a combination of both. Unfortunately, none of these methods accurately indicates the amount of resources (both direct and indirect) consumed in the provision of services. Logically, the consumption of resources and corresponding productivity levels are closely related. One could argue that a practice's charges are indicative of the resources consumed, but is that really true? Are a practice's charges based on resources consumed (i.e., are they actually cost based)? Most group practices today would probably have to admit that they are not. Some groups would argue that their charges are market based, but exactly what does that mean? Most likely it means that charges for the new year are based on what they were last year, plus some minor percentage increase to cover inflation. There is a better way of tracking productivity: RVUs.

RVUs are nationally standardized, thus they can be used for clinical productivity and cost benchmarking. Currently, RVUs are also the best measurements available that are statistically valid (they measure what they purport to measure) and reliable (repeated measurements yield the same results). RVUs are also interpretable, feasible to collect, based on a representative sample and sensitive to change when variation exists. RVUs also relate to cases resulting in high volume, cost, risk or profile.

Caution should be used when utilizing only RVUs to measure productivity. Other important measures include "good citizenship" or community work, quality and outcomes of care, administrative duties and collegiality, teamwork, peer review, academic teaching and research, and overall satisfaction of the patients, staff and providers. Measures of quality are just as important as measures of quantity in analyzing productivity, so include both subjective and objective measures in the final mix.

Keep in mind that not all data are good data. They must be both statistically valid and reliable to earn the trust of those using the data to propagate change. It is critical to first learn how to interpret and fully understand the numbers before sharing them with others. Use data analysis first as an informational tool before implementing it as an educational tool—it will take time for physicians and other clinical providers to learn to trust what the data are telling them. Remember that data are quantitative tools that may cause irreparable damage if used to judge others. "Be gentle" with them.

DISCUSSION
Proper Coding Is Critical to RVU Analyses

Proper coding is critical to accurate RVU analyses. Inaccurate coding results in a variety of problems, not the least of which can lead to an audit and major penalties. If a medical practice does not code properly for its procedures and services, it affects the charges, third-party payer reimbursements, and productivity and cost analyses. It will also trickle down to eventually affect provider compensation if the physicians and/or nonphysician providers are paid based on charges, productivity and/or RVUs. If the coding is inaccurate, the data will not be accurate for RVU analyses. It's that simple.

A study of family practice physicians observed patterns of undercoding and overcoding.[1,2] In general, the results showed that the physicians were fairly accurate in their coding, but that there were certain situations resulting in either an under- or overvaluation of the visit. Researchers in this study found that undercoding was more likely when the visit was longer and involved less focus on treatment, when it resulted in a referral or when the patient was a child. Overcoding was more likely to occur with shorter, more social, or less complicated visits, when the visit focused on prevention or treatment and when a medical student was present. Overcoding also occurred more frequently when no referral was made and no drugs were prescribed. Oddly enough, this study also found that visits with patients who had fee-for-service insurance were more likely to be coded accurately.

An article in the August 2001 edition of the *Physician Profiling and Behavior Change Report* gave some good tips for working with physicians on proper coding. Tommy H. Smith, executive administrator and chief financial officer for Rocky Mount Family Medical Center (NC), was interviewed about his approach to proper coding. He gives his providers reports on a regular basis to help them track their own individual productivity and compare it to the group's goals. Coding reports are given to the physicians weekly, so that any tweaking needed can be taken care of immediately. Smith notes that "when you give physicians good data, they tend to improve performance on their own. Ninety percent of the time, if a physician's RVU performance slips, I get copied on an e-mail asking if other physicians have advice on how to deal with no-shows or how to code a certain procedure." He goes on to state that "new physicians tend to undercode."[3]

Undercoding and/or overcoding are not the only pitfalls that need to be avoided. Lisa Stavrakas, a senior consultant with the MGMA Health Care Consulting Group, provides an example. Most general surgeons miss coding for the mesh used when performing incision hernia repairs. CPT code 49561 (repair initial incision or ventral hernia; incarcerated) has work RVUs of 14.25, but they can also bill for CPT 49568 (implantation of mesh) with work RVUs of 4.89. Most surgeons only code for the 49561 but forget the mesh. Mesh can only be coded in addition to incision or ventral hernia repairs. That's where certified coders, who catch such details, earn their keep.

Training on coding for physicians is important because, while they receive minimal or no coding education during their years of medical school and residency, they are financially and legally responsible for correctly reporting the codes used for the services they deliver.

This author's recommendation is that physicians receive on-site or in-house training for several reasons:

- The clinic loses productivity, revenue and the cost for sending physicians to off-site training sessions. It is more cost effective for the clinic to hire and pay travel expenses for a coding expert to come to the practice to conduct an on-site training session;
- On-site training provides an opportunity for all of the physicians at that clinic to attend the training; and
- An on-site trainer ensures that all of the physicians at that clinic are receiving the same training information rather than attending different training sessions and receiving different information.

Leanne Travers, a consultant with Gold Consulting Group, notes that there are some situations, such as OB/Gyn, where groups have large contracts with global delivery fees. Practices are recording the patient visit in the medical records, but an encounter sheet is not filled because the patient is a global case. Therefore, the visit and the CPT codes are not recorded in the practice management/billing system. Groups need to record every visit and all services provided at the time of care for several reasons:

- Patients vary in the amount and type of care they require. If the group serves a patient population that presents more complicated cases where the cost of care provided exceeds the fee paid, then it needs to record and document for the next contract negotiations;

- If no encounter form is filled out, those "fee-for-service" exceptions in most global contracts could be lost and the revenue not collected;
- All services should be recorded so that workload comparisons among providers can be analyzed; and
- If all CPT codes are not documented, it cannot be determined whether the cost of care exceeds income derived from individual contracts or from the group as a whole.

DISCUSSION
Modifiers

Modifiers are used, among other things, to adjust the reimbursement of a service or procedure to account for assistant surgeons, multiple procedures, bilateral procedures, etc. If the reimbursement is adjusted for a CPT code, it would be logical that the charge and associated RVUs would be similarly affected. Most medical procedure modifiers (with the primary exception of anesthesia codes) make adjustments by percentages rather than amounts.

If a CPT-4 code has a modifier attached, be sure to note the effect of that modifier on the associated charge because you will need to adjust the total RVUs for that code in the same manner. For example, if a modifier reduces a procedure's charge by 50 percent, the *total* RVUs (not just the work or practice expense RVUs) for that procedure with the modifier need to be reduced by 50 percent. If the RVUs are not adjusted, the productivity and cost for that procedure are distorted, and the analyses will yield inaccurate results.

It was mentioned in chapter 1 that the TC (technical component) modifier indicates that the practice is billing only for the technical component. The 26 modifier indicates that the practice is billing only for the professional component. The reason that some codes (usually for radiology and pathology) are listed three times in the RBRVS is for reporting either the global service (both technical and professional components), just the technical component or just the professional component. Listing a code three times like this allows each part of the service to be billed.

For example: CPT code 71020 (radiologic examination of the chest with both frontal and lateral views) without a modifier indicates that the clinic is billing for both the technical component and the professional component. CPT code 71020-TC indicates that the clinic is billing for the technical component ONLY. In this case the clinic probably owns the X-ray machine, so internal staff takes the film and then sends out the film to be read. CPT code 71020-26 indicates that the clinic is billing for the professional component ONLY, meaning that the radiologist interprets and documents on the film. A multispecialty clinic that owns its X-ray machine and an employed radiologist that interprets the films would bill code 71020 (no modifier), taking and reading the film. A multispecialty clinic that owns its X-ray machine and sends the films out to a separate radiologist would bill code 71020-TC for taking the film. A radiology practice that receives films from the multispecialty clinic would bill code 71020-26 for reading the film. The same process holds true for the pathologist reviewing a biopsy specimen.

Exhibit 2.1 lists some of the more common Medicare modifiers and provides an example of the effects those modifiers have on the total RVUs for a given procedure.

RVUs vs. Encounters

Studies have consistently shown that the most important predictor of the total amount of work involved in a patient's visit is not the number of encounters but rather the *time* involved with each encounter.[4,5] That's why RVUs are more effective than encounters for tracking productivity. RVUs take into consideration the time and intensity of visits, whereas encounters simply count the number of visits.

An encounter is defined by the Medical Group Management Association as a documented, face-to-face contact between a patient and a provider who exercises independent judgment in the provision of services to the individual. If the patient with one diagnosis sees two different providers on the same day, the visits

EXHIBIT 2.1. Modifier Effects on RVUs

Modifier	Description	Adjustment to RVUs
–50	bilateral procedure	1.5
–51	multiple procedure	0.5
–62	co-surgeon	0.625
–78	return to OR related procedure	0.5
–80 to –82	surgical assistant	0.16

Example for CPT 61458, excise skull for brain wound:

CPT/ Modifier	Description	Adjustment	Adjusted RVUs
61458		0	48.46
61458-50	bilateral procedure	1.5	72.69
61458-51	multiple procedures	0.5	24.23
61458-62	co-surgeon	0.625	30.29
61458-78	return to OR	0.5	24.23
61458-80	surgical assistant	0.16	7.75

are counted as one encounter. If the patient sees two different providers on the same day for two different diagnoses, these visits are considered two encounters. An encounter as defined by the MGMA *Physician Compensation and Production Survey Report* includes only procedures from the evaluation and management chapter (CPT codes 99201-99499) or the medicine chapter (CPT codes 90800-99199) of the *Physician's Current Procedural Terminology,* fourth edition, copyrighted by the American Medical Association.

Prior to the introduction of RVUs, medical groups had no quantitative means for tracking provider productivity except through simply counting the number of procedures performed and patients seen (visits or encounters). Within families of codes, such as the outpatient office visit codes for new and established patients, administrators could also compare coding patterns to other groups and physicians, but that offered little beyond simple volume measures. RVUs greatly expanded the possibilities to allow for analysis of case complexity and mix, staffing and workload, procedure cost, productivity-based compensation models, etc.

As an introductory way of looking at the difference between RVUs and encounters, let's say there are two piles of coins on a table, each representing one encounter per coin. Each pile contains 10 coins, so each pile represents 10 encounters. So far, the piles appear to be equivalent in value. However, as we take a closer look, we see that one pile has only copper pennies, while the other has a mix of silver coins. Which pile has more value? The pile of pennies is obviously of less value than the pile of silver coins. Without RVUs, encounters are little more than tick marks of productivity. They are pennies that will not increase in value. With RVUs and encounters combined, one can count productivity or value in not only the number of procedures (number of coins), but also in the relative value assigned to each procedure (denomination of each coin).

Exhibit 2.2 demonstrates the relative differences between established patient office visit codes. Each of the office visits constitutes a count of one, giving the appearance that the same amount of time and effort was involved in each visit. To the contrary, it is impossible to ascertain the variance in the consumption of resources involved in the provision of any particular office visit without using relative value units. Relative to CPT-4 code 99212 with a total RVU of 1.00 (RBRVS 2002 values), 99214 with a total RVU of 2.18 takes more than twice the amount of time and effort. It's easy to see in this exhibit why it is important to track RVUs as well as encounters when tracking workload. Remember that total RVUs encompass time, effort, resources consumed and the risk involved in the provision of a clinical service. When strictly analyzing the work component, the only elements involved are time and effort (and skill, of course, which is inherent in the type of service being provided).

As a further exploration of the difference in using RVUs vs. encounters, Exhibit 2.3 displays encounter and RVU_w information

THE EYES HAVE IT

Eye is a term used to describe the way herding dogs control livestock with their gaze. Border Collies have an *intense eye*; Aussies are considered *loose-* to *medium-eyed* dogs, usually focusing on a group rather than an individual animal. His breed notwithstanding, NERO, an Aussie from the Midwest, uses an intense eye at his first sight of the Atlantic.

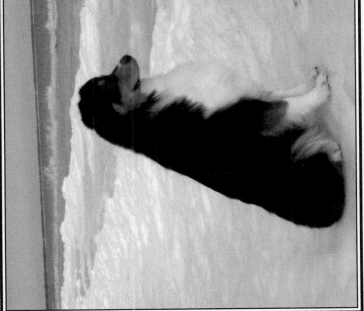

NERO (AUSTRALIAN SHEPHERD).—BETH RICE, PECULIAR, MO

EXHIBIT 2.2. Relative Differences Between Office Visit Codes

CPT-4	Description	RVU_w	RVU_{pe}	RVU_m	Total RVU	Encounter
99212	Office visit	0.45	0.53	0.02	1.00	1
99213	Office visit	0.67	0.69	0.03	1.39	1
99214	Office visit	1.10	1.04	0.04	2.18	1

for four family practice physicians. As a rule, the RVU_w component rather than the total RVU is used in measuring provider productivity. This component is used because the work component is specifically designed to measure a medical provider's skill and effort as well as the degree of decision-making complexity required for performing a procedure. The other rule to keep in mind is that the higher the RVU value, the higher the procedure complexity and the higher the resource consumption for delivering services.

Exhibit 2.3 is also a classic example that demonstrates the invaluable information that a practice administrator gains from performing a provider productivity analysis that combines CPT code frequency and RVU data.

The first observation is that Doctor 4 has the highest number of office visits; however, Doctor 2 has the highest RVU_w productivity. This observation indicates three potential questions and/or problems for the administrator to explore. The first issue is that Doctor 4 is serving a high number of patients whose medical issues are less complex, thus the practice is underutilizing Doctor 4. The second issue is that Doctor 4 is undercoding services and/or providing incomplete documentation of services. The third issue involves whether or not Doctor 4 is assigned to a walk-in clinic and/or patient triage.

The second observation is that all four doctors most frequently use code 99201 for new patient office visits and 99212 for established patients. For example, typical coding patterns for a family of codes such as this would generally follow a normal or bell-shaped curve, i.e., most of the visits should fall in the middle of the curve or around code 99203 for new patient visits and 99213 for established patient visits. All four physicians are coding at the low end of the range for new patient and established patient visits; therefore, the data indicate a severe coding problem. Not only are the physicians understating the services that they are providing, they are also understating RVU productivity and resources that are actually consumed in the provision of services. So why is this important? According to the American Association of Health Plans *Annual Industry Survey*, 1998, 56.3 percent of third-party payers, excluding Medicare and Medicaid plans, calculate their physician fee schedules based on the RBRVS and therefore on a set dollar amount per RVU called the conversion factor. As a result,

EXHIBIT 2.3. Provider Productivity Analysis

Code	2002 RVUw	Dr. 1 Office Visits	Dr. 1 RVUw	Dr. 2 Office Visits	Dr. 2 RVUw	Dr. 3 Office Visits	Dr. 3 RVUw	Dr. 4 Office Visits	Dr. 4 RVUw
99201	0.45	3	1.35	33	14.85	75	33.80	210	94.50
99202	0.88	2	1.76	29	25.52	22	19.40	35	30.80
99203	1.34		0.00	44	58.96	29	38.90	24	32.20
99204	2.00	1	2.00	18	36.00	32	64.00	9	18.00
99205	2.67		0.00	10	26.70		0.00	1	2.70
99211	0.17	400	68.00	191	32.47	386	65.60	41	7.00
99212	0.45	1,835	825.75	1,986	893.70	2,329	1,048.10	2,329	1,048.10
99213	0.67	459	307.53	711	476.37	727	487.10	29	19.40
99214	1.10	221	243.10	248	272.80	185	203.50	162	178.20
99215	1.77	14	24.78	24	42.48	9	15.90	22	38.90
Totals:		**3,122**	**3,651.71**	**4,463**	**5,427.70**	**4,231**	**5,030.24**	**4,708**	**5,296.39**
Difference:			**529.71**		**964.70**		**799.24**		**588.39**

Note: Some office visit codes are not shown, but are included in totals.

undercoding is actually minimizing revenue and practice cash flow. This will be discussed in more detail in chapter 4 on managed care contracting.

The third observation is that on average Doctor 1 is producing 31 percent less RVUs than his or her colleagues. There are several possible explanations. Perhaps Doctor 1 is new to the practice and therefore has less available data and fewer patients than the other physicians. Another scenario is that the doctor may be retiring soon and is reducing the time to see patients, especially new patient visits. Or, perhaps Doctor 1 instructed the appointment scheduling staff that he or she wants to stop seeing new patients. Whatever the case may be, the practice administrator needs to use this type of information for determining the reason for the low productivity in relation to the other three providers.

Exhibits 2.2 and 2.3 both clearly illustrate the invaluable, objective information that practice administrators gain when combining CPT code frequency and RVU data for assessing provider productivity. It is imperative that administrators trust their data and use the information to learn more about their practices. Data analysis is a valuable ally that helps administrators identify potential productivity problems before they have a serious effect on practice performance.

RVUs vs. Fees

Unless a practice's charges are cost based instead of historically based, the charges are a poor indication of resources consumed in the provision of services. Charges can be easily manipulated to reflect discounts, charity care and third-party payer reimbursements. Without tracking the resources consumed, how can a practice accurately track productivity besides counting the number of office visit codes billed out? Historical-based fees are really arbitrarily and/or subjectively determined. The use of RVUs in tracking productivity provides a nonmonetary, objective method that is not subject to sliding fee scales. Another aspect to consider is that fees vary a considerable amount geographically, while RVUs, which are universal, remain constant.

RVUs and Staffing

RVUs can also be used to justify staffing needs within an organization. Let's say that one of your branch administrators has been requesting additional support staff for his or her busy practice. At first glance, during a review of the total procedure volume and charges for the providers in that particular office, neither measure has increased much over the past year.

To better understand the situation, you should look at productivity for the providers in that clinic. Set up a spreadsheet that contains the CPT codes billed out by that clinic for each of the last two or three years and that shows the frequency (or total count) of each of those codes. Next, sort by frequency in descending order. Multiply the work RVUs by the code frequency to attain the total work output as measured in RVUs. Look at the differences in both the types of codes and the total work RVUs for each year. Is there an observable change in E&M coding?

Perhaps the group is seeing an increase in the number of new patients, who take more time to evaluate and therefore have higher RVUs than established patients. If the RVUs have increased by 20 percent or more, it may indicate a change in case complexity or patient mix. This change may be enough to warrant additional staff to handle the increase in time spent with each new patient or with the more complicated cases. (*Note:* One could also use total RVUs instead of only work RVUs. This author chose to use work RVUs because they were stable over the last few years compared to the malpractice and practice expense components, which were converting to resource-based values, and therefore in flux.)

FTE Providers

A brief discussion of full-time equivalent (FTE) providers is necessary for an understanding of how the denominator for some calculations is reached. RVUs strictly measure clinical productivity, so a clinical FTE (or CFTE) needs to be defined. A detailed discussion is provided in the sidebar, but, briefly, the CFTE provider is defined by the number of clinical hours the practice considers to be the minimum for a normal clinical workweek. Clinical work includes time the provider devotes to patient care and supporting activities.

When comparing productivity among providers who work a different number of hours each month or who have administrative, research, or teaching duties mixed with clinical time, it is important to use the FTE or CFTE designation in the denominator. It makes any comparison equitable by converting the clinical productivity time into a full-time equivalent standard rather than analyzing it on a per person basis.

DISCUSSION
Full-Time Equivalent (FTE)

According to MGMA, an FTE physician or nonphysician provider works whatever number of hours the practice considers to be the minimum for a normal workweek, which could be 37.5, 40, 50 hours or some other standard. To compute the FTE of a part-time provider, divide the total hours worked by the provider by the number of hours that your medical practice considers being a normal work week. Note that some practices have a different standard number of hours for physicians than for nonphysician providers. For example, a provider working in a clinic or hospital on behalf of the practice for 30 hours compared to a normal workweek of 40 hours would be 0.75 FTE (30 divided by 40 hours). A provider working full time for three months during a year would be 0.25 FTE (3 divided by 12 months). A medical director devoting 50 percent effort to clinical activity would be 0.50 FTE. Do not report a provider as more than 1.00 (i.e., 100 percent) FTE, regardless of the number of hours worked. The MGMA *Cost Survey Report* includes in this category practice physicians such as shareholders/partners, salaried associates, employed and contracted physicians and locum tenens; residents and fellows working at the practice; and only physicians involved in clinical care. Not included are full-time physician administrators. The FTEs are totalled for whatever specific category is requested. These categories may include the practice (employees and providers); providers (both physicians and nonphysician providers); or physicians (only those providers with an academic degree designation of doctor of medicine [MD], doctor of osteopathy [DO], doctor of dental surgery [DDS], or doctor of pediactric medicine [DPM]). This sum is not the total number of people, but the total FTEs.

In a medical school setting, department faculty FTE includes faculty compensated by the department with a minimum rank of instructor and an academic degree designation of MD, DO, MD/PhD or PhD, regardless of duties performed within the department (for example, clinical, research, teaching or administration).

Clinical FTE

A clinical FTE (CFTE) provider is defined by the minimum number of *clinical hours* the practice considers to be the minimum for a normal *clinical workweek. Clinical work* includes time during which the provider devotes to patient care and supporting activities, i.e. medical records update, consultation with other providers, preparation for clinical and/or surgical procedures, patient phone contact, etc. Non-clinical activities, such as teaching, research, writing and administration, should be excluded from CFTE calculation. In some cases, full-time equivalency may be the same as *clinical* full-time equivalency. CFTE can never be greater than 1.00, regardless of the number of hours worked. Provider-assigned duties, such as administrative responsibilities, research, etc., are not included as clinical work. To calculate CFTE, the number of clinical hours worked is divided by the number of total hours worked in a normal workweek. For example, a provider who performs 20 hours of clinical work, 10 hours of administrative work, and 10 hours of research in a practice where the normal week is 40 hours is considered 1.00 FTE and 0.50 CFTE (20 divided by 40 hours).

A resident CFTE is defined by the rotations completed in the reporting period. A resident is considered 1.0 CFTE if all 12 months are spent at the home institution. If a resident spends fewer than 12 months, the CFTE is determined by dividing the number of months spent at the home institution by 12. For example, a resident spending nine months at the home institution and three months on rotation at a private clinic or fulfilling research requirements is counted as 0.75 CFTE (9 divided by 12 months). Use the sum of only the clinical FTEs for physicians and/or nonphysician providers. This sum is not the number of physicians and/or nonphysician providers, but the total FTE for *clinical work* only.

In a medical school setting the CFTE is the sum of the clinical FTEs for all full-time and part-time compensated faculty members. Voluntary faculty FTEs are not included.

Note the inherent problem with this method if using FTE or CFTE in external comparisons. If each group has a different number of standard clinical work hours per week, it is difficult at best to attempt to benchmark against other practices. For benchmark purposes, it would be better to report the number of hours worked per week and the number of weeks worked per year; that way, vacations, continuing medical education (CME) time, sick time, leaves of absence, etc., would not interfere with the measurement of clinical productivity and subsequent comparisons of that activity.

PRODUCTIVITY CASE STUDY

A group practice has the following specialties and FTE providers: Internal Medicine—3.75 FTE, Family Practice—4.00 FTE, Obstetrics/Gynecology—1.00 FTE and Pediatrics—2.00 FTE. The CEO wants a complete productivity analysis including the specialties and each of the providers within those specialties. As an initial step we obtained all the necessary data to create the following tables. We used our practice management billing system to obtain the total charges, total procedures and total patients for six months. To obtain the RVU values, we used the *Federal Register* that contained the RBRVS issued by the Department of Health and Human Services (HHS), and we matched the RVU value to the CPT codes that were billed out of our clinic during the same time period. The RVU value was then multiplied by the CPT code frequency and summed to obtain a total RVU for the group. Now let's take a closer look at the data to see what observations can be made about this group practice.

Group/Specialty Summary Reports

To analyze the data, we start by reviewing the group level and specialty level summary reports' key indicators as shown in Table 2.1, and then drill down to the provider level. For this case study, we will utilize the year-to-date (YTD) average for six months of data. (In your practice you may want to perform an analysis based on current month, quarter or annual data.) Begin by highlighting the highest and lowest numbers in each category, and by comparing each specialty to the group level indicators. Any numbers that raise questions will need to be further investigated. For further explanation of the key indicators, please refer to the glossary at the back of this book.

At first glance, one area that stands out is that the OB/GYN providers are completing the fewest procedures (Procedures/FTE) with a six-month median of 2,014. However, they have by far the highest charge per procedure (Charge/Procedure) of $175.01 and the highest charge per patient (Charge/Patient) of $232.80. Does this make sense for this particular specialty practice? If we look closer, we also notice that the per OB/GYN providers have the highest RVUs per patient, and their RVUs per procedure are more than three times higher than the other specialties. Both of these RVU ratios measure case complexity. This tells us that even though these providers are performing fewer procedures, they are performing more complicated procedures, and their charges should reflect this. So far so good.

The pediatric group appears to be managing the least complicated patients (shown by RVUs/Patient), but it is averaging the second highest charge per FTE. This may seem to be a problem, but we can also see that the pediatric group is averaging a higher number of procedures per FTE than any other specialty. This measure tells us that, even though the pediatricians are performing less complicated procedures, they are making up for it with volume. They are also charging the most for their services (Charge/RVUs). We may need to make adjustments to the internal fee schedule. Another angle of analysis is to look at the types of procedures billed by each physician. A high volume of procedures in a managed care environment (especially a capitated environment) is normally not a good thing. We need to make sure that quality and not quantity is the rule of thumb for decision making by each physician.

The internal medicine group also has several numbers that stand out on the table. This group is producing the lowest charge per procedure, indicating either an undercoding problem or a

TABLE 2.1. Group Practice Productivity Analysis by Specialty

Ratios	YTD Averages for Six Months				
	Group	Internal Medicine	Family Practice	OB/GYN	Pediatrics
Charge/Procedure	$58.95	$45.15	$56.07	$175.01	$53.58
Charge/Patient	$90.51	$69.40	$88.34	$232.80	$81.71
Procedure/Patient	1.50	1.50	1.60	1.30	1.50
Procedures/FTE	3,217	2,960	3,463	2,014	3,806
Charge/FTE	$189,602	$133,656	$194,166	$352,462	$203,943
RVUs/Procedure	1.24	1.06	1.14	3.55	1.06
RVUs/FTE	3,975	3,136	3,948	7,141	4,020
RVUs/Patient	1.90	1.63	1.80	4.72	1.61
Charge/RVU	$47.70	$42.62	$49.18	$49.36	$50.73

need to review the internal fee schedule for this primary care specialty. The group is also producing the lowest number of RVUs per FTE, which may be another indication of undercoding that needs to be investigated further by reviewing each CPT code billed out by each provider and comparing it to the medical charts. Since the internal medicine group is the lowest producing specialty in most of the categories, we need to further investigate what is happening within this particular specialty.

We can also analyze the type of services the specialties are providing by looking at specific code ranges. If we look at the percentage of total RVUs earned in each range, we can evaluate if the providers are spending their time providing the right types of services. Looking at Table 2.2, how would one know if the services provided look reasonable for each specialty? Note that E&M codes fall between 99201 and 99499, and surgery codes number from 10040 to 69990. "Medicine" as used in the table means medical services falling between CPT codes 90281 and 99199. Immunizations fall within the medicine code range.

It appears that these specialties are providing the right types of services. Most of the time you will know by simply thinking about the types of procedures each specialty performs. One would expect that OB/GYN would have a high volume of surgical codes, and pediatrics would have a very low volume within that same code range. If some of the numbers seem high, the next step would be to look at the individual codes billed for each code range. The internal medicine group providers are spending most of their time conducting office visits and little time doing minor surgery. The family practice providers are splitting their time between office visits and the surgery room, while the OB/GYN physicians are spending the majority of their time delivering babies. The pediatricians are also spending a large part of their time with office visits, but they also have the highest percentage of medicine codes.

For more detail, we can take a look at the top codes that are billed out of the group practice for each specialty. This will allow us to start looking in detail at the types of services the specialties are providing. This kind of detail can be expanded to include more codes; but for the purpose of this case study we will look at

TABLE 2.2. Types of Services Provided by Specialty

Services	Group	Internal Medicine	Family Practice	OB/GYN	Pediatrics
		Percentage of Total RVUs Earned in Each Range			
E&M (99201–99499)	68.36	82.94	59.24	30.92	80.98
Surgery (10040–69990)	24.09	9.13	34.43	68.03	7.27
Medicine (90281–99199)	7.55	7.93	6.33	1.05	11.75

the top three codes utilized in each section range by specialty and their frequency (count) of utilization in each of three categories.

Looking at the detail in Table 2.3, we see that the top E&M code for most of the specialties is 99213. The internal medicine group has 99212 as its top E&M code. This is an indication of either undercoding or having a larger population of less complicated patient diagnoses. In either situation, the coding suggests that we need to further investigate what is happening in the internal medicine group.

In the surgery range, all of the specialties are using 36415 (drawing blood) as their top code. If we look at family practice, the next two most frequently used codes are 59410 (obstetrical care) and 59025 (fetal non-stress test). The clinic currently employs only one full-time OB/GYN provider. If the family practice group is performing these types of procedures, would it be of benefit to hire another OB/GYN provider to take over these cases? To answer that question, we would also need to review the cost data to determine the overall feasibility of hiring another OB/GYN physician or perhaps a nonphysician provider.

In the medicine section range, it appears that the specialties are performing as expected. The pediatric group is utilizing the codes in this range the most, followed by internal medicine, then family practice and finally OB/GYN. The top three pediatrics codes (90700, 90782 and 90648) are all vaccine-related injections, which are expected given a pediatrician's patient population.

Specialty/Provider Summary Reports

After analyzing the group and specialty summary information and the specialty detail reports, we can further investigate the specialties that raised questions for us by drilling down to the next level of detail. In this example, we will look more closely at the physicians in internal medicine. Table 2.4 compares the data for the internal medicine physicians to that of other providers in the practice as a whole. We can start reviewing the data by highlighting the highest and lowest performers in each category.

Looking at the providers in internal medicine, Dr. Michaels stands out as the lowest producing provider in several categories. Dr. Michaels has performed the fewest number of procedures

TABLE 2.3. Top Codes Utilized in Each Section Range by Specialty

Internal Medicine (FTE = 3.75)

	CPT	Count	CPT	Count	CPT	Count
E&M	99212	3,566	99213	2,859	99214	1,101
Surgery	36415	1,987	69210	130	10060	24
Medicine	90718	543	93000	245	90782	187

Family Practice (FTE = 4.00)

	CPT	Count	CPT	Count	CPT	Count
E&M	99213	4,259	99212	2,994	99214	1,634
Surgery	36415	1,878	59410	527	59025	213
Medicine	90718	363	90780	191	90700	149

OB/GYN (FTE = 1.00)

	CPT	Count	CPT	Count	CPT	Count
E&M	99213	889	99212	536	99395	82
Surgery	36415	244	57454	60	59410	55
Medicine	90782	28	90784	20	93000	17

Pediatrics (FTE = 2.00)

	CPT	Count	CPT	Count	CPT	Count
E&M	99213	3,230	99212	1,563	99391	287
Surgery	36415	784	17110	62	69210	34
Medicine	90700	727	90782	208	90648	188

TABLE 2.4. Analysis of Internal Medicine Providers

Ratios	Internal Medicine	YTD Average for Six Months				
		Dr. Nelson	Dr. Michaels	Dr. More	Dr. Itall	
Charge/Procedure	$45.15	$47.79	$37.23	$49.65	$45.91	
Charge/Patient	$69.40	$71.22	$74.86	$70.25	$61.27	
Procedures/Patient	1.50	1.50	1.80	1.60	1.10	
Procedures/FTE	2,960	3,358	2,362	3,251	2,869	
Charge/FTE	$133,656	$161,375	$85,178	$169,559	$118,512	
RVUs/Procedure	1.06	1.09	.96	1.26	.93	
RVUs/FTE	3,136	3,471	2,392	3,574	3,107	
RVUs/Patient	1.63	1.65	1.86	1.67	1.34	
Charge/RVU	$42.62	$42.60	$39.92	$42.01	$45.93	

(Procedures/FTE), produced the smallest amount of charges (Charge/FTE) and produced the least amount of RVUs (RVUs/FTE). We will need to gather more information to understand why Dr. Michaels is producing at a level so far below his peers.

Drs. More and Nelson are the top performing providers within this specialty. Their numbers are very close to each other, and they are both producing better than the internal medicine average. For now, we will keep them on the same pace, but we'll also continue to monitor their progress.

Although not the least productive provider, Dr. Itall is performing a significantly fewer number of procedures than the two top performing providers. Dr. Itall is also accumulating fewer charges and fewer RVUs than Drs. Nelson and More. To determine what is happening with these two providers, we can take closer look at the services and procedures they are billing. This can help us evaluate the service mix and can give us a first look at the coding habits of each provider.

Provider Procedure Detail

Finally, we can drill down in the analysis to look at the codes each provider is billing to get a better idea of what type of caseload each has. We can then better understand the reasons behind their productivity levels. Table 2.5 shows the four internal medicine doctors and their most frequently used codes in each of the section ranges that we are analyzing. Again, this kind of detail can be expanded to include more codes, but for the purpose of this case study we will look at the top three codes and their frequency (count) of utilization in each of three categories.

We can see from the table that Drs. Nelson and More both have 99213 as their top E&M code. However, Drs. Michaels and Itall both have 99212 as their top code. If we were to graph their code frequency, we would see that neither Dr. Michaels nor Dr. Itall follow the normal bell-shaped curve for the E&M code range. This could be caused by a high frequency of less complicated patient diagnoses or a possible undercoding issue. To determine the reasons, we would need to do a chart audit to verify coding compliance and determine if coding education is necessary within the department.

TABLE 2.5. Top Codes Utilized in Each Section Range by Internal Medicine Providers

Dr. Nelson	CPT Count	CPT Count	CPT Count
E&M	99213 – 863	99214 – 692	99212 – 489
Surgery	36415 – 783	29075 – 16	54150 – 10
Medicine	90718 – 150	93000 – 83	90700 – 74

Dr. Michaels	CPT Count	CPT Count	CPT Count
E&M	99212 – 735	99213 – 564	99202 – 171
Surgery	36415 – 422	None	None
Medicine	90718 – 92	93000 – 66	90707 – 45

Dr. More	CPT Count	CPT Count	CPT Count
E&M	99213 – 842	99212 – 764	99214 – 469
Surgery	36415 – 731	69210 – 32	20610 – 11
Medicine	90718 – 121	90732 – 75	93000 – 52

Dr. Itall	CPT Count	CPT Count	CPT Count
E&M	99212 – 1,208	99213 – 528	99214 – 265
Surgery	36415 – 481	10060 – 15	11200 – 10
Medicine	90782 – 84	90718 – 52	93000 – 44

We also can see that Dr. Michaels is the only provider that has a new patient code (99202) in the top three codes. Are the internal medicine group providers seeing new patients, or have they closed their practices to new patients? This could be another reason for the overall low productivity of this specialty compared to the group. We may want to investigate these questions further by expanding our analysis to look at the frequency and graph the curve of all the office visit codes (CPT codes 99201 to 99205 for new patients and 99211 to 99215 for established patients). This can be a useful tool to help providers visualize coding issues. Further recommendations are discussed below.

Case Study Conclusions

After reviewing our productivity analysis reports, we conclude that our specialties' productivity levels are relatively consistent to those of their respective professions. The internal medicine specialty is the lowest producing of the four. We decided to do a more in-depth analysis of the internal medicine doctors' productivity for assessing individual provider productivity efficiency.

The following observations were made for each internal medicine physician:

1. Dr. Nelson has the second highest productivity with an RVU total of 3,471 for this six-month period. All key indicators are reasonable for internal medicine. An analysis of her top three CPT codes utilized for each section range indicates that she is seeing very complex patient conditions. Considering that Dr. Nelson's second-most-frequently billed E&M code is 99214, it is suggested that a chart audit be conducted to confirm this observation and to verify that she is not overcoding.

2. Dr. Michaels is the lowest producer among the internists. He produced only 2,392 RVUs. Further investigation found that he has just started with the group and is in the process of building a practice. An analysis of his top three CPT codes utilized for each section range indicates that he is seeing more new patients than the other physicians as

evidenced by CPT 99202, the third-most-frequently billed E&M code. A concern that should be investigated is that his highest CPT code is 99212. This indicates a high probability that he is undercoding office visits. We may want to conduct a chart coding audit for estimating any potential lost clinic revenue and to correct any coding errors so that the practice remains in compliance.

3. Dr. More's productivity is the highest of his peers with an RVU total of 3,574. One concern is that the E&M code frequencies for 99213 and 99212 are very close. This indicates a probability that undercoding is occurring for office visits. We may want to conduct a chart-coding audit for estimating any potential lost clinic revenue.

4. Dr. Itall's productivity is the third highest within this specialty. Her RVU total is only 3,107. An analysis of this provider's top three frequently used CPT codes for each section range confirms a severe undercoding issue. In this case the most frequent CPT code is 99212, used 680 more times than her second code 99213. Data such as these warrant conducting an extensive chart-coding audit in order to stop clinic revenue loss.

For the internal medicine group, we conclude that there is a need to conduct an extensive chart-coding audit to check for coding compliance and loss of revenue to the clinic. We also recommend that the group be required to attend a coding seminar to emphasize the importance of correct coding practices. We will continue to monitor the internal medicine group, as well as the rest of the specialties, and will reevaluate their progress six months from now.

Key Productivity Indicators

Neither RVUs nor any other single ratio or figure should be used as the solitary indicator of provider productivity. There are a number of key practice management indicators that should be used in combination to give a complete picture of each provider's productivity level and workload within the office.

Case intensity and trends in patient population can be measured using a combination of encounters, RVUs and procedures per patient. Procedure complexity, an indication of case intensity, is measured through the number of RVUs per procedure.

Workload, office volume and staffing requirements can be measured using a combination of encounters, RVUs, procedures and patients per FTE provider. It is also helpful to separately measure the nonphysician providers from the physicians to gain an understanding of how the workload is divided. Finally, periodically review the composition of the top volume codes to determine changes in practice trends and treatment protocols. Notice that none of these key indicators includes charges (or fees) as either a numerator or denominator. Charges are too subjective in most cases to be used as an accurate measure of productivity.

CONCLUSION

Prior to the introduction of RVUs, medical groups had no quantitative means for tracking provider productivity except through simply counting the number of procedures performed and patients seen. The introduction of RVUs provided an objective and equitable measure of clinical productivity, but they should not be used as the sole measurement because of extraneous variables such as administrative work, research, teaching, community work, etc. Use RVUs as part of the overall, balanced scheme of tracking productivity.

Notes

1. Chao, J., Gillanders, WR., Goodwin, MA., Stange, KC. (1998). Billing for Physician Services: A Comparison of Actual Billing with CPT Codes Assigned by Direct Observation. Journal of Family Practice 47:28.32.
2. Kikano, GE., Chao, J., Gotler, RS., Stange, KC. (1999, Nov/Dec). Identifying Patterns of Over- and Under-coding. Family Practice Management 6(10): 12–13.
3. Use These Simple Formats to Develop Financial Profiles. (2001, August). Physician Profiling & Behavior Change Report 4(8):113–118.

4. Hsiao, WC., Braun, P., Dunn, D., Becker, ER., Yntema, D., Verrilli, DK., Stamenovic, E., Chen, S. (1992, November). An Overview of the Development and Refinement of the Resource-Based Relative Value Scale, Medical Care, 30(11) Supplement.
5. Lasker, RD., Marquis, MS. (1999). The Intensity of Physicians' Work in Patient Visits. New England Journal of Medicine 341(5):337–341.

CHAPTER **3**

RVU Cost Analysis

INTRODUCTION

In recent years the interest in RVU cost analysis has been on the rise. Why all the excitement? Revenues minus costs equal the bottom line of any business, including the business of health care. The bottom line sets the standard of living for clinicians and staff, and no one wants to lower his or her standard of living. Health care reimbursements have been declining over the past decade due in part to managed care and third-party payer reimbursements; therefore, medical organizations must be cognizant of the financial health of their practices and be proactive in managing it.

RVU cost analysis places the knowledge, and therefore the power, in the hands of the administrator to negotiate revenues and analyze expenditures. Cost analysis at the per-unit level allows for procedure profitability (or loss) analysis, setting internal fee schedules based on costs, contract negotiation based on RVU cost and utilization, equitable provider compensation packages based on productivity and overhead coverage, and the tracking of ancillary and referral utilization risks. In short, RVU cost accounting uses the RBRVS instead of stopwatches and clipboards.

Even if your practice has a software or Internet-based program that calculates the cost per procedure for you and performs all types of analyses, it is important to realize how those costs are calculated so that you can fully comprehend where the numbers come from. You know that your physicians will be asking you for the calculations and for the formulas for exactly how the figures were derived, so be ready with the answers!

Measuring Costs

Like productivity, cost has been measured numerous ways over the years. Articles on this topic have some duplication of cost indicators, but each list is slightly different due in part to the sheer number of possibilities. For example, those cost indicators listed include length of hospital stay, cost per visit, cost per covered life in managed care plans, cost reduction as a part of net revenue, expenditures per RVU, nonemergent emergency room visits, cost per FTE provider, etc.

There are several key indicators used when measuring costs in RVU analysis. The blended cost per RVU is the foundation for all other cost-per-RVU analyses. It is used for internal purposes as a comparison of volume to cost control and for third-party payer contract negotiations. The blended cost per RVU can be split into RVU component costs, as we'll see in the RVU Cost Accounting 101 section that follows.

Building on the cost per RVU concept, the cost per procedure can be compared to reimbursement per procedure from third-party payers and/or to the practice's charge per procedure. From there, a cost-based fee schedule can be set with a little buffer built in for profitability and bad debts.

Cost per provider is an important indicator for those practices that compensate their physicians and nonphysician providers based on productivity and overhead coverage. If a medical practice has more than one specialty, the expenses should probably be allocated per specialty. Consumption of overhead resources can vary considerably depending on the specialty (for example, family practice vs. OB/GYN), so an equitable division and allocation of those expenses can drastically affect the cost per unit.

RVU Cost Accounting 101

Cost accounting determines the cost per unit of a product or service. For medical groups, RVU cost accounting determines the cost per *relative* unit of services rendered. Units of measure (in this case, relative value units) recognize relative differences in resources consumed through the production of goods and services. Each unit receives a similar amount of cost.

To calculate the cost per RVU, divide the total practice costs by the total RVUs billed out during a given time period, typically year-to-date. The expense and time periods must match. Cost per RVU is the cornerstone of all RVU cost analyses. It is an indication of the cost control vs. volume within a group practice. The formula is as follows (note that Σ [Greek letter for 'sigma'] means "sum"):

$$\frac{\Sigma \text{ Total expenses}}{\Sigma \text{ Total RVUs}} = \text{Cost/RVU}_{\text{blended}}$$

Although this concept will be covered in greater detail later in the chapter, it is important to point out from the beginning what is included in total costs. From an administrator's point of view, physician compensation is part of the total cost in the operation of a medical practice; if you ask the physicians, they would say that their compensation would not be considered a practice cost. From this author's viewpoint, *total costs* means *total costs including everyone's compensation.* After all, physician compensation is money and benefits paid to the physicians; it is not revenue. It is money that is going out of the practice, not coming in—therefore, it is an expense and a cost to the practice. Despite the differences in opinions, CMS recognizes that one of the three components in the RBRVS is "physician." If the government can recognize compensation as an expense or cost, then shouldn't the rest of the health care field?

It is important to note that overstating RVUs results in understating the cost per RVU, thus accurate coding is critical to the success of any RVU analysis. For a brief (and elementary) example, let's say total costs equal $100. If the total RVUs are 20, then the cost per RVU (total costs divided by total RVUs) is $5. If, on the other hand, total RVUs were inaccurately reported as 25, then the cost per RVU would show as $4.

This blended cost per RVU is also the bottom line for contract negotiation based on RVUs and conversion factors. A conversion factor is simply the dollar amount paid per RVU by third-party payers. It converts RVUs into money for reimbursement of medical procedures. If the practice accepts a conversion factor that is lower than its blended cost per RVU, it will lose money on every procedure billed to that insurance carrier. For example, let's say that a given practice has a blended cost per RVU of $50. Conversion factors from Payer #1 and #2 are $49 and $50.50 respectively. Exhibit 3.1 shows the cost per procedure to this particular group practice compared to the money lost or gained per procedure based on these two conversion factors. This is not to say that a practice should decline all contracts that offer a conversion factor below the practice's bottom line figure. Negotiation should include consideration of the overall volume generated by a given contract and the proportion of total practice revenue expected from the contract. In other words, make decisions based on the big picture, not on one particular scenario.

COST/RVU$_W$

Component cost per RVU is also useful for the practice to calculate and analyze. The cost per work RVU (denoted as RVU$_w$) is calculated by dividing the sum of the total provider compensation by the sum of the total work RVUs. The result is what the practice is, on average, paying its providers per work RVU.

$$\frac{\Sigma \text{ Total provider compensation expenses}}{\Sigma \text{ Total RVU}_w} = \text{Cost/RVU}_w$$

The next logical question to answer is "What comprises total provider compensation expenses?" Should both nonphysician providers and physicians be included? If so, what are the criteria for inclusion/exclusion? What expenses should be included or excluded using what criteria? These are all very important questions that deserve some thought because there are now no national standards. Currently there are three schools of thought regarding these questions that for simplicity's sake we'll call Theory #1, Theory #2 and Theory #3. Think of each theory as part of a continuum.

At the far end of the continuum is Theory #1. The premise of this theory is that only physicians' straight salary should be included in the provider compensation expense because that was the logic used when the RBRVS was created. Keeping in mind that the RBRVS was created a decade ago and that, at the time, nonphysician providers were not utilized at the level they are now, there is some merit to this approach. For example, let's say the

EXHIBIT 3.1. Costs Per Procedure Based on Payer Conversion Factors

CPT Code	Description	RVU$_{total}$	Cost	Payer #1	Payer #2
99201	Office/outpatient visit, new	0.93	$46.50	$45.57	$46.97
99202	Office/outpatient visit, new	1.67	$83.50	$81.85	$84.34
99203	Office/outpatient visit, new	2.50	$125.00	$122.50	$126.25
99204	Office/outpatient visit, new	3.60	$180.00	$176.00	$181.80
99205	Office/outpatient visit, new	4.56	$228.00	$223.44	$230.28
99211	Office/outpatient visit, est	0.55	$27.50	$26.95	$27.78
99212	Office/outpatient visit, est	0.98	$49.00	$48.02	$49.49
99213	Office/outpatient visit, est	1.37	$68.50	$67.13	$69.19
99214	Office/outpatient visit, est	2.16	$108.00	$105.84	$109.08
99215	Office/outpatient visit, est	3.16	$158.00	$154.84	$159.58

Conversion factors: Payer #1 = $49.00, Payer #2 = $50.50

physicians are paid on a strict contract salary, and their benefits and any bonuses are taken from the operation's profits. The only thing the practice pays in bad times would be the physician's contract salary amount. That means that each physician is responsible for his or her own insurance, retirement, etc. When times are good, the physician could receive that money from the practice to make those payments, but when times are bad, the funds come out of his or her own pocket. For most group practices now, however, this approach is much too simplistic to be realistic or competitive in the market.

Theory #2 is a middle-of-the-road approach. If the nonphysician providers each bill out for their own clinical services using their own unique provider identification numbers, then these providers and their compensation should be included as part of the provider compensation expense along with physicians and their compensation. If they do not bill out for their own services, then their expenses are part of the general practice expenses, such as overhead.

What components of the nonphysician and/or physician compensation should be included or excluded under Theory #2? This theory promotes standardization of these expenses, so think about what is included in any basic compensation package. It would include straight salary, employee payroll taxes (FICA/Medicare, federal unemployment and state unemployment), basic insurance (health, dental, life, disability and worker's compensation) and the defined retirement plan. Everything else would be included with overhead expenses. While this theory offers standardization for comparison and benchmarking, it does not give the practice its true cost per work RVU.

Examples of these account categories taken from the *Chart of Accounts for Health Care Organizations*, published in 1999 by the MGMA Center for Research in Ambulatory Health Care Administration, are displayed in Table 3.1. Similar account categories are available for nonphysician providers. Table 3.1 is not meant to be a definitive model; it merely offers the suggestion of what could be included. Not every medical practice will need a chart of accounts structure this detailed.

TABLE 3.1. Detailed Expense Categories

Account Number	Description
8000	**PROVIDER-RELATED EXPENSES**
8100	**PHYSICIANS—SALARIES**
8110	Salaries, Distributions and Incentives (Physician)
8120	Salaries—Owner/Stockholder (Physician)
8130	Distribution and Incentives (Physician)
8140	Global/Capitation Distributions (Physician)
8150	Employee Salaries (Physician)
8160	Employee Incentives (Physician)
8170	Administrative Salaries (Physician)
8180	Other Compensation (Physician)
8200	**PHYSICIAN—EMPLOYEE-RELATED EXPENSES**
8210	Payroll Taxes (Physician)
8211	Payroll Taxes—FICA/Medicare (Physician)
8212	Payroll Taxes—Federal Unemployment Insurance (Physician)
8213	Payroll Taxes—State Unemployment Insurance (Physician)
8214	Payroll Taxes—Other (Physician)
8220	Insurance (Physician)
8221	Insurance—Health (Physician)
8222	Insurance—Dental (Physician)
8223	Insurance—Life (Physician)
8224	Insurance—Disability (Physician)
8225	Insurance—Workers' Compensation (Physician)
8226	Insurance—Other (Physician)
8227	Insurance—Officers' Life (Physician)
8230	Pension and Retirement Benefits (Physician)
8231	Pension (Physician)
8232	Deferred Compensation (Physician)
8233	Severance Plan (Physician)
8235	Professional Development (Physician)
8240	Books and Subscriptions Physician)
8245	Dues and Memberships (Physician)
8250	Licenses (Physician)
8255	Meetings (Physician)

(continued)

continued
TABLE 3.1. Detailed Expense Categories

Account Number	Description
8260	Travel (Physician)
8265	Medical Reimbursement Plan (Physician)
8270	Vehicles (Physician)
8271	Leased Motor Vehicles (Physician)
8275	Parking (Physician)
8280	Telephone (Physician)
8285	Beepers (Physician)
8290	Meals and Entertainment (Physician)
8295	Other Benefits (Physician)

Theory #3 is the other end of the continuum. Like Theory #2 it includes both physicians and nonphysician providers who bill for their own clinical services using their own unique provider identification codes. It also includes all direct expenses (except malpractice insurance premiums, which are assigned their own category of expense). Ask yourself, "But for this provider, would we incur this expense?" If the answer is "no," then the cost is considered a direct expense and should be included in the total provider compensation expenses. This means all discretionary income is included in the cost per work RVU, which gives the practice a much truer picture of its costs and what it is paying providers (on average) per work RVU. Discretionary income includes salaries, distributions, incentives, bonuses, payroll taxes, insurance, pension and retirement benefits, professional development, books and subscriptions, dues and memberships, licenses, meetings, travel, medical reimbursement plans, vehicles, parking, telephones, beepers, meals and entertainment, etc. Any compensation-type expense that can be linked directly to a particular physician and/or nonphysician provider would be included in the total provider compensation. Table 3.2 displays the categories included from the *Chart of Accounts for Health Care Organizations*. Again, similar categories and accounts are available for nonphysician providers.

Keep in mind that it is not always as cut-and-dried as this example in every situation. Practices may use nonphysician

TABLE 3.2. Provider-Related Expenses

Account Number	Description
8100	**PHYSICIANS—SALARIES**
8150	Employee Salaries (Physician)
8200	**PHYSICIAN—EMPLOYEE-RELATED EXPENSES**
8210	Payroll Taxes (Physician)
8211	Payroll Taxes—FICA/Medicare (Physician)
8212	Payroll Taxes—Federal Unemployment Insurance (Physician)
8213	Payroll Taxes—State Unemployment Insurance (Physician)
8214	Payroll Taxes—Other (Physician)
8220	Insurance (Physician)
8221	Insurance—Health (Physician)
8222	Insurance—Dental (Physician)
8223	Insurance—Life (Physician)
8224	Insurance—Disability (Physician)
8225	Insurance—Workers' Compensation (Physician)
8230	Pension and Retirement Benefits (Physician)

providers in a variety of ways. In some instances, the nurse practitioner or physician assistant will provide independent service for which they can bill directly; however, in other instances, they may provide services in place of the physician, for which they cannot bill independently. Examples include telephone triage. The problem according to Leonard J. Lichtenfeld, MD, member of the RBRVS Update Committee, is that "it is sometimes difficult to know how to apportion the salaries of these providers: as a practice expense, or a compensation expense. If a nurse does just independent stuff or all 'incident to' stuff, there is no question; but, if his/her activities are a mix, then it can become confusing."

This problem also relates to practice expense and Medicare. If groups determine their practice expenses with respect to Medicare reimbursement, they can calculate how much of the fee payment is allocated to "practice expense." If they don't correctly allocate the practice expense of a nurse, they may inflate the practice expense side of the equation. If they compare how much Medicare pays for "practice expense" and find their "practice expense/RVU" is much greater than Medicare's reimbursement, they may say it doesn't pay to take Medicare—but they may ignore the fact that the non-physician provider may also be billing directly, which is an "income generator."

Dr. Lichtenfeld goes on to say, "As you can see, this is very complicated and it may be beyond anyone's practical compre-hension. But it also points out the problems in trying to properly allocate expenses. Maybe the right way is to determine the pro-portion of time a nurse spends in independent vs. incident-to activities, and then allocate their costs appropriately. For example, I have a nurse practitioner who sees patients on her own 3/10 ses-sions weekly. The rest of the time she helps me triage phone calls, contacts patients regarding lab results, schedules surgery, etc. So, 30 percent of her salary/benefits would be on the compensation side of the ledger, and 70 percent would be on the practice expense side."

COST/RVU$_{PE}$

The cost per practice expense RVU (denoted as RVU_{pe}) is cal-culated by dividing the sum of the total practice expenses (over-head) by the sum of the total practice expense RVUs. Practice managers should monitor this figure when keeping an eye on the costs and volume within each cost center.

$$\frac{\Sigma \text{ Total practice expenses}}{\Sigma \text{ Total RVU}_{pe}} = \text{Cost/RVU}_{pe}$$

Depending on the theory adopted by a practice, once the provider compensation and the malpractice expense issues are taken care of, it's easy to calculate what goes into the practice expense component: everything left over related to operating expenses. If nonphysician providers are not included as part of the provider compensation expense, then all their expenses are considered part of overhead. Other expense categories include salaries and fringe benefits for ancillary staff and employees, informational systems, office and administrative supplies, billing and clinical supplies, occupancy, cost of goods sold (medical relat-ed), purchased services/management fees and some nonoperating expenses such as interest and income tax expense.

COST/RVU$_M$

The cost per malpractice RVU (denoted as RVU$_m$) is calculated by dividing the sum of the total malpractice premium expense by the total malpractice RVUs. This figure is simply the cost of malpractice coverage per RVU. (This calculation does not apply to Federally Qualified Health Centers [FQHCs] that don't pay malpractice premiums due to coverage by the Federal Tort Claims Act. In that case all malpractice RVUs would be left out of all RVU analyses.)

$$\frac{\Sigma \text{ Total malpractice expenses}}{\Sigma \text{ Total RVU}_m} = \text{Cost/RVU}_m$$

This expense includes the total malpractice insurance premiums paid for physicians and, depending on the theory adopted, perhaps for nonphysician providers. If the nonphysician providers bill out for their own clinical services using their own unique provider identification numbers, and if their compensation expenses are included as part of the total provider compensation expense, then their malpractice premiums should be included in this separate category of total malpractice expense. If nonphysician provider expenses are included as part of overhead, then their malpractice premiums should also be included as part of the practice's overhead.

Data Required for Calculations

To calculate the practice's cost per RVU you will need a spreadsheet package (such as Excel^{TM}), the RBRVS (it can be downloaded off the CMS Web site free of charge, since it is a public use file, available at www.cms.gov), your practice expenses discussed above and a productivity report (sorted preferably by provider). There are several RBRVS files from which to choose on the CMS Web site. Download the Excel^{TM} file with the CPT codes, descriptions and RVUs. Exhibit 3.2 gives an example of how the RBRVS file appears. There are several different columns with information extraneous to the RVU discussions in this book. In this book we will use the HCPCS (column A), modifier (column B), description (column C), work RVU (column F), fully implemented nonfacility practice expense RVU (column G), malpractice RVU (column J), and fully

EXHIBIT 3.2. RBRVS File

2002 National Physician Fee Schedule Relative Value File

CPT codes and descriptions only are copyright 2001 American Medical Association. All Rights Reserved. Applicable FARS/DFARS Apply.

Dental codes (D codes) are copyright 1994 American Dental Association. All Rights Reserved.

Released 11/1/2001

	HCPCS	mod	Description	Work RVU	Fully Implemented Nonfacility PE RVU	MP RVU	Fully Implemented Nonfacility Total
2612	10040		Acne surgery	1.18	1.00	0.05	2.23
2613	10060		Drainage of skin abscess	1.17	1.51	0.08	2.76
2614	10061		Drainage of skin abscess	2.40	1.88	0.17	4.45
12146	99201		Office/outpatient visit, new	0.45	0.47	0.02	0.94
12147	99202		Office/outpatient visit, new	0.88	0.77	0.05	1.70
12148	99203		Office/outpatient visit, new	1.34	1.12	0.08	2.54
12149	99204		Office/outpatient visit, new	2.00	1.51	0.10	3.61
12150	99205		Office/outpatient visit, new	2.67	1.80	0.12	4.59
12151	99211		Office/outpatient visit, est	0.17	0.38	0.01	0.56
12152	99212		Office/outpatient visit, est	0.45	0.53	0.02	1.00
12153	99213		Office/outpatient visit, est	0.67	0.69	0.03	1.39
12154	99214		Office/outpatient visit, est	1.10	1.04	0.04	2.18
12155	99215		Office/outpatient visit, est	1.77	1.36	0.07	3.20

implemented nonfacility total RVUs (column K). For descriptions of the other column indicators plus the columns not visible on Exhibit 3.2, consult the current year's fee schedule as published in the *Federal Register.*

The time period for the analysis is typically year-to-date with the expense period matching the productivity period. In addition to the total group expenses, be sure to break out the costs by component (work, practice expense and malpractice). The reasoning behind the year-to-date approach to cost analysis is that it is easier to match expenses and productivity if it is done year-to-date rather than by plucking a month or quarter out of the year. Also, practice expenses can fluctuate wildly from one month to another, so it usually does not make sense to perform a cost analysis on anything *but* year-to-date. In addition, there may be year-end expenses that affect the cost per RVU and that wouldn't show up in mid-year analyses. In general, this type of cost analysis is performed on either an annual or semi-annual basis only—rarely more frequently due to the time involved relative to the report value. If your group has extra time and resources to put into this type of analysis, you may wish to conduct it more often.

The productivity report will come from the billing system. Ideally, the report will include every CPT-4 code and its frequency billed out *by provider,* both with and without modifiers, the charge per procedure and the total charges. It's important to list the productivity (clinical procedures billed) by each physician and each nonphysician provider, so that both productivity and cost analyses can be performed at the provider level. Including the procedure charges allows comparisons between the cost and the charge per procedure.

If a CPT-4 code has a modifier attached, be sure to note the effect of that modifier on the associated charge because you will need to adjust the total RVUs for that code in the same manner. For example, if a modifier reduces a procedure's charge by 50 percent, the *total* RVUs (not just the work or practice expense RVUs) for that procedure with the modifier need to be reduced by 50 percent. If the RVUs are not adjusted, the productivity and cost for that procedure are overstated, and the analyses will yield inaccurate results.

Exhibit 3.3 displays the information discussed in this section. Obviously you will need to merge the data from the productivity

EXHIBIT 3.3. Productivity Report Merged with RBRVS File

	A CPT	B mod	C Description	D MD ID	E freq	F total charge	H total RVUw	J total RVUpe	L total RVUm	M total RVU
2	10040		Acne surgery	188	2	$56	2.36	2	0.1	4.46
3	10040	52	Acne surgery	188	33	$417	19.47	16.5	0.825	36.795
4	10060		Drainage of skin abscess	25	2	$91	2.34	2.3	0.16	4.8
5	10060		Drainage of skin abscess	94	1	$40	1.17	1.15	0.08	2.4
6	10060		Drainage of skin abscess	110	3	$176	3.51	3.45	0.24	7.2
7	10060		Drainage of skin abscess	120	1	$65	1.17	1.15	0.08	2.4
8	10060		Drainage of skin abscess	188	10	$537	11.7	11.5	0.8	24
9	10060	52	Drainage of skin abscess	188	2	$67	1.17	1.15	0.08	2.4
10	10060		Drainage of skin abscess	359	1	$63	1.17	1.15	0.08	2.4
11	10060	52	Drainage of skin abscess	359	1	$50	0.585	0.575	0.04	1.2
12	10060		Drainage of skin abscess	370	3	$253	3.51	3.45	0.24	7.2
13	10060		Drainage of skin abscess	379	9	$426	10.53	10.35	0.72	21.6
14	10060	52	Drainage of skin abscess	379	1	$50	0.585	0.575	0.04	1.2
15	10060		Drainage of skin abscess	398	5	$284	5.85	5.75	0.4	12
16	10060		Drainage of skin abscess	819	2	$126	2.34	2.3	0.16	4.8
17	10060		Drainage of skin abscess	824	3	$189	3.51	3.45	0.24	7.2

report with the RBRVS file. How you do that will depend on the reporting capabilities of the billing system. Exhibit 3.3 is a very small portion of the resulting spreadsheet. Note that the work, practice expense, malpractice and total RVUs are frequency adjusted and that the providers are listed by ID number only and not by name. Also note that the modifier –52 reduces each of the RVU components by half.

Estimating RVUs

Estimating RVUs for those procedures that do not have RVUs assigned is not difficult, but it can be time consuming. If a particular code does not constitute a material portion of the business performed, it is probably OK to leave it out of the analysis and not bother with the RVU estimation. Note that RVU estimation is not intended as a method for assigning values to all the pathology, laboratory and HCPCS codes. Those codes and procedures are not assigned values in the RBRVS for a reason: CMS reimburses pathology and lab procedures on a flat fee basis. In CMS's view, HCPCS codes are subsumed within the medical procedures associated with them and therefore do not require their own RVUs.

The first step when estimating RVUs is to separate the procedures (CPT-4 codes) and their corresponding charges into section ranges by code category. In general, a good method of categorizing the code ranges is by using the AMA sections described in its annual CPT books and displayed in Table 3.3. Note that the HCPCS codes are not listed here. Remember that HCPCS codes were

TABLE 3.3. Section Ranges by Code Category

Section	Code Range
Evaluation and Management	99201 to 99499
Anesthesiology	00100 to 01999, 99100 to 99140
Surgery	10040 to 69990
Radiology	70010 to 79999
Pathology and Laboratory	80049 to 89399
Medicine (except anesthesiology)	90281 to 99199

developed by CMS for its own Medicare reimbursement purposes, thus they are not part of the CPT listing developed by the AMA.

The logic behind this basic categorization is that charges and RVUs tend to be similar within the same range of codes. Naturally the code ranges would have to be much smaller than these broad categories in order for this logic to bear itself out, but the framework is now in place. Within some of these code ranges are what are sometimes referred to as "families of codes," which vary in complexity (and therefore RVUs), but are all centered on a certain procedure or service. For example, there are five different CPT-4 codes for outpatient office visits for established patients (99211 to 99215). This small range of codes could be considered a "family" because they all involve the same type of service, but require different levels of time and complexity and, therefore, are assigned different RVUs.

Now that the section ranges are set up, within each range calculate (A) the average charge per procedure for those procedures with a zero RVU. Next, within that same section range, calculate (B) the average charge *per RVU* per procedure for each code with non-zero RVUs. Finally, divide (A) by (B) to arrive at (C) an estimated RVU. The example of this calculation in Exhibit 3.4 is purely fictitious and is used for illustration purposes only.

Remember that this exercise simply provides a means of estimating the *cost* of providing services that do not have RVUs assigned through the RBRVS. Most medical practices do not include lab, pathology or HCPCS codes when tracking clinical productivity, for several reasons. First, a staff member who is not a physician, physician assistant or nurse practitioner typically provides these procedures and services. Clinical productivity is tracked only for those providers who bill out for their own services using their own unique provider ID codes (for example, MDs, DOs, PAs, and NPs). Second, there is no work component calculated using this methodology. It is assumed that the costs associated with the provision of these services are practice expenses (overhead).

Exercise caution if using this methodology to estimate entire section ranges of codes. If possible, use an entire year's worth of data or more to estimate values because the specific codes used

---

EXHIBIT 3.4. Calculation of Estimated RVUs

A = average charge per procedure with zero RVUs within a code range
CPT 20936 = $75/procedure

B = average charge per RVU per procedure with RVUs within the same code range
CPT 20937 = $100 procedure/5.89 total RVUs
= $16.98 per RVU
CPT 20938 = $125 procedure/6.37 total RVUs
= $19.62 per RVU
Sum = $36.60
Average charge = $36.60/2 = $18.30

C = A/B = 75/18.30 = 4.10 RVUs for CPT 20936

---

and the charges associated with each code may vary considerably from one period to the next. If values are assigned to a wide variety of codes using charge and RVU data from just a few codes, the results will vary each month. Using as many codes as possible will lessen the chance of wide fluctuation over time. It will also help to limit the range of codes to families of codes when estimating values.

Before any RVU estimations are finalized for a given procedure, it may be a good idea to get input and buy-in from the clinicians. Ask them about the relative difficulty of the procedure and the time, skill and resources required for that code compared to a similar code with established RVUs.

You may wonder why you can't just use the McGraw-Hill *Relative Values for Physicians* (RVP) for the pathology and lab code ranges. After all, that particular scale has values assigned to each category, so what's the problem? The primary concern is the effect of mixing different scales. Remember that the McGraw-Hill scale comprises five independent scales, so values are relative to each other only within a given category and not across the entire CPT code range. If the RBRVS and McGraw-Hill scales are mixed and

RVP values from pathology and lab codes are thrown in for comparison and costing purposes, then any analysis is fundamentally invalid. Stick with one scale or the other, but don't mix and match!

Cost per RVU Calculations

First, on a spreadsheet like that shown in Exhibit 3.5, arrange the data from the billing system (sorted by CPT code then by individual providers using their billing identification codes). Then, enter the RVUs from the RBRVS file and multiply the procedure count by each RVU component (work, practice expense and malpractice) to determine total RVUs. The last column is the total RVUs generated for each code by frequency and clinician. The last row gives the totals for each RVU component. Exhibit 3.5 shows an example of office visit encounters for some physicians in a multispecialty group practice. Even though this example lists only office visit codes, the concept applies to all CPT codes billed by a practice's clinicians during a given time period.

If a given CPT code does not have RVUs assigned in the RBRVS file, calculate the RVUs for it using the formula provided in Exhibit 3.4, and enter those total RVUs into the empty cells for that code. The use of estimated RVUs for tracking provider productivity of HCPCS codes is not recommended, but a practice can use them to estimate the costs associated with the provision of those services. The practice of breaking out the estimated RVU total into components is also not recommended, especially if HCPCS are the codes with the estimated RVUs. HCPCS codes are typically termed nonprofessional services; therefore, the physician work component is not relevant. If a practice insists on breaking out the RVUs for HCPCS, realize that close to 100 percent of the total RVUs belong in the practice expense category. The only exception to that is the proportion of the total RVU associated with malpractice coverage. For simplicity in this exercise, just plug in the total RVUs and multiply the total by the code frequency.

Now that the total RVUs have been calculated for each component and the total, the figures can be plugged into the cost per RVU formulas discussed earlier. Using fictional numbers for both

EXHIBIT 3.5. Total RVU Components for Office Visit Encounters

	A CPT	B mod	C Description	D MD ID	E freg	F total charge	H total RVUw*	J total RVUpe*	L total RVUm*	M total RVU*
2266	99201		Office/outpatient visit, new	94	304	$13,175	136.8	142.88	6.08	285.76
2269	99201		Office/outpatient visit, new	110	312	$13,200	140.4	146.64	6.24	293.28
2297	99202		Office/outpatient visit, new	370	29	$1,816	25.52	22.33	1.45	49.3
2298	99202	52	Office/outpatient visit, new	370	273	$14,360	120.12	105.105	6.825	232.05
2323	99204		Office/outpatient visit, new	94	358	$39,331	716	540.58	35.8	1292.38
2386	99212		Office/outpatient visit, est	120	4263	$151,646	1918.35	2259.39	85.26	4263
2388	99212		Office/outpatient visit, est	131	2132	$77,061	959.4	1129.96	42.64	2132
2413	99213		Office/outpatient visit, est	25	357	$20,030	239.19	246.33	10.71	496.23
2414	99213	52	Office/outpatient visit, est	25	50	$2,341	16.75	17.25	0.75	34.75
2443	99213		Office/outpatient visit, est	824	1028	$57,452	688.76	709.32	30.84	1428.92
2464	99214		Office/outpatient visit, est	379	185	$17,120	203.5	192.4	7.4	403.3
2477	99215		Office/outpatient visit, est	110	43	$5,016	76.11	58.48	3.01	137.6
2478	99215		Office/outpatient visit, est	120	29	$2,985	51.33	39.44	2.03	92.8
2936	Totals:**						61933.9	60327.775	6850.115	129111.79

2937 *NOTE: 2002 RBRVS non-facility values multiplied by count

2938 **Not all rows are shown, but are included in totals

the numerators and denominators, the formulas provide the following results:

Cost/RVU$_w$

$$\frac{\Sigma \text{ Total provider compensation expenses}}{\Sigma \text{ Total RVU}_w} \quad \frac{\$195,454.29}{5325.73} = \$36.70$$

Cost/RVU$_{pe}$

$$\frac{\Sigma \text{ Total practice expenses}}{\Sigma \text{ Total RVU}_{pe}} \quad \frac{\$236,068.59}{5702.14} = \$41.40$$

Cost/RVU$_m$

$$\frac{\Sigma \text{ Total malpractice expenses}}{\Sigma \text{ Total RVU}_m} \quad \frac{\$3,604.49}{236.36} = \$15.25$$

Cost/RVU$_{blended}$

$$\frac{\Sigma \text{ Total expenses}}{\Sigma \text{ Total RVUs}} \quad \frac{\$435,127.37}{11264.23} = \$38.63$$

Why don't the individual component figures add up to the blended cost per RVU figure? The answer is that different denominators are used in each calculation.

In analyzing the results, one may wonder if these figures fall within a normal range of costs, or if the figures are out of line. Benchmarking will answer these questions. One of the most common reports cited when comparing notes with other ambulatory care practices is the MGMA *Cost Survey Report,* which calculates both the cost per RVU$_w$ and the cost per RVU$_{blended}$. Obviously the per unit costs will vary, depending on the methodology applied to the categorization of costs previously discussed. This should be noted when comparing any practice's costs to another practice's costs, especially when attempting to benchmark against another practice.

Cost per Procedure Calculations

There are two basic methods used to calculate a cost per procedure for any given CPT code. One way is to lump the components together (that is, using the blended cost per RVU); the other method splits the total RVUs into individual RVU components. Both methods are valid, and each will give slightly different results. Consistency in the methodology used is key. Using the previous cost per RVU figures, the "lump" method for CPT code 99213 is calculated as follows:

$$RVU_{total} * Cost/RVU_{blended} = \text{procedure cost}$$

$$1.37 * 38.63 = \$52.92$$

Some administrators prefer to break out the components in order to examine each component's contribution to the total cost. The "splitter" method is calculated like this:

$$(RVU_w * Cost/RVU_w) + (RVU_{pe} * Cost/RVU_{pe}) + (RVU_m * Cost/RVU_m) = \text{procedure cost}$$

$$(0.67 * 36.70) + (0.67 * 41.40) + (0.03 * 15.25) =$$

$$24.589 + 27.738 + 0.4575 = \$52.78$$

The malpractice cost of CPT code 99213 for this particular imaginary practice is 46 cents, the overhead cost is approximately $27.75 and the provider cost is slightly less than $24.60.

Cost-Based Fee Schedules

Until recently, many of the ambulatory health care practices based the charge for any given procedure on two primary drivers: its historical charge and its market-based charge, (that is, what the competition down the street charged). In addition, a few medical practices set their fees based on what the insurance carriers would pay for a service. Some calculated an average charge based on what various survey results showed for fee ranges.[1] It is important to note that survey reports simply state how practices price certain procedures, not how the procedure *should* be priced.

When setting fees for the upcoming year, administrators looked at what their practice charged for a procedure during the past year, and then maybe increased the fee a bit to what they believed the market would bear. Before any changes were made to the fee, however, they would cleverly have a staff person anonymously call the competition and pretend to be a potential patient who was inquiring what their fee was for the same procedure. That way the administrator could adjust the group's fees to remain competitive, regardless of whether or not the gross charges covered practice expenses. If that sounds like price fixing or a violation of current antitrust laws, you're correct. It was indeed flirting on the fringes of it. Today, doing anything that would give the mere impression that two or more medical practices have conferred and/or agreed upon pricing may warrant an investigation (read: trouble) from the Department of Justice.

In the "old days," any or all of these methods may have had some merit (even if pricing errors and biases were perpetuated) because there was no superior alternative. Does the same logic apply in today's markets? After all, they are practicing *medicine* so traditional business protocol does not apply to their operations, right? Wrong!

If a medical practice does not set a cost-based fee schedule and work to ensure that the revenue generated covers its costs, it will not remain financially viable. Medical practices no longer have the luxury of pretending that business rules do not apply to them. They must face the fact that they are in the *business* of medicine and the organization needs to be run just like any other business. For better or for worse, the advent of managed care forever changed the face of ambulatory health care administration.

So how would a practice revise its fee schedule to become cost-based? It's actually fairly simple. Determine the cost for each procedure and add a percentage on top of it to act as a buffer against discounts and bad debts. The "cost-plus" amount now becomes the practice's standard fee for that procedure.

Comparing Costs to Charges

Questions often heard from practice administrators are "What are our top 20 codes in terms of total costs?" and "Are we covering our costs on those codes?" Savvy administrators know the 80/20 rule applies to health care as much as it does to other industries. Twenty percent of the codes comprise 80 percent of the total volume, so why look at all the codes when a few will do?

Exhibit 3.6 provides a simple format and hypothetical example for this particular analysis. For this exercise you will need a spreadsheet with the following data: CPT codes billed out for the time period under analysis, any modifiers billed out with those codes, brief descriptions of the CPT codes (helpful but not manda-

EXHIBIT 3.6. Analysis of Costs-to-Charges for Top Codes

	cpt	mod	des	freq	cost/proc	total cost	gross chg	disc chg	variance
	A	B	C	D	E	F	G	H	I
2	99213		Office/outpatient visit, est	12,210	63.07	770,140.66	982,133	687,493	-82,648
3	99203		Office/outpatient visit, new	5,185	114.68	594,596.08	631,714	442,200	-152,396
4	27447		Total knee replacement	221	2,459.28	543,499.90	1,344,342	941,039	397,539
5	99212		Office/outpatient visit, est	9,514	45.58	433,618.54	549,884	384,919	-48,700
6	99214		Office/outpatient visit, est	4,069	96.18	391,354.78	540,538	378,377	-12,978
7	99202		Office/outpatient visit, new	3,380	82.11	277,539.55	285,577	199,904	-77,636
8	20610		Drain/inject joint/bursa	3,265	83.74	273,399.16	304,496	213,147	-60,252
9	29881		Knee arthroscopy/surgery	290	909.94	263,883.66	786,071	550,250	286,366
10	22612		Lumbar spine fusion	113	2,265.72	256,026.37	664,052	464,836	208,810
11	63030		Low back disk surgery	182	1,381.09	251,358.81	769,278	538,495	287,136
12	27130		Total hip replacement	107	2,314.47	247,648.60	672,235	470,565	222,916
13	99204		Office/outpatient visit, new	1,277	167.94	214,458.15	213,414	149,390	-65,068
14	22554		Neck spine fusion	89	2,083.47	185,428.56	406,761	284,733	99,304
15	29888		Knee arthroscopy/surgery	114	1,604.00	182,855.68	574,853	402,397	219,541
16	27244		Repair of thigh fracture	95	1,770.78	168,223.91	305,425	213,798	45,574
17	23420		Repair of shoulder	99	1,541.21	152,579.57	441,127	308,789	156,209
18	99213	25	Office/outpatient visit, est	2,307	63.08	145,514.90	185,875	130,113	-15,402
19	72100		X-ray exam of lower spine	2,583	54.63	141,121.02	259,909	181,936	40,815
20	99455		Disability examination	890	138.35	123,128.72	160,734	112,514	-10,615
21								total variance	1,438,516

tory), frequency of utilization per CPT code, the cost per CPT code and the gross charge per procedure. Multiply the frequency by the cost per procedure to get the total cost, then sort the data in descending order by total cost. Now you can carve out the top 20 codes by total cost and proceed with the exercise. Multiply the frequency by the gross charge per procedure (not shown in Exhibit 3.6) to get the total gross charges. In turn, multiply the total gross charge per procedure by the average discount per procedure (in this example a 30 percent discount was used) to derive the total discounted charge per procedure (column H). Next, subtract the total discounted charge (column H) by the total cost (column F) per procedure to get the variance (or profit or loss) per procedure.

Why look at net charges (or discounted charges) instead of gross charges? Because it is more reasonable to look at what the practice anticipates in revenue generation rather than gross charges that no one pays.

As you can see by this particular example, some procedures are profitable while others are not. If the fee schedule (gross charges) is cost-based with an added buffer for profit, the result should reflect a profit on every procedure. In reality the discount varies by procedure, and rarely would a flat discount rate (30 percent in this example) apply across all CPT code categories. When performing this exercise, you will want to apply the appropriate average discount (which will vary by payer) to each procedure range. E&M codes may have one discount, for example, while surgery codes may have another typical discount off gross charges.

Comparing Costs to Reimbursements

There are a couple of different methods to use when comparing your practice's costs to various reimbursements. Two of the more common methodologies compare costs to reimbursements based on a factor of the RBRVS and to reimbursements based on a conversion factor. Both are discussed below.

Reimbursements Using a Factor of RBRVS

A fictitious medical specialty practice used to compensate its physicians and nonphysician providers based upon net productivity. Historically, the practice measured clinical work performed by the total RVUs and total gross charges billed. Over the last several years, however, gross charges have become less valid, as various payers want billing based on contractual arrangements for reimbursement. It's time to educate the clinicians on a new compensation strategy using RVUs, which will be the new measure of productivity that replaces gross charges. As part of the overall billing system change, the group is restructuring its fee schedule to convert it to a factor of the RBRVS since that is what the major insurance carriers are using as the basis of their fee reimbursements.

The illustration in Exhibit 3.7 calculates the factor by dividing the cost per procedure by the Medicare fee schedule per procedure. The factor per code is multiplied by the code frequency to obtain the adjusted factor. Finally, the frequency-adjusted factor (column G) is divided by the frequency (column F) to derive the blended, overall rate reflecting cost as a factor of the RBRVS (1.13 in this case).

This information should prompt the administrator to do two things: (1) raise the group's own internal fee schedule by a minimum of 14 percent to cover costs and (2) renegotiate third-party payer contracts to cover those costs. Some contractors base reimbursements on a factor of the RBRVS, so this group would be wise not to accept anything lower than 113 percent of the Medicare rate.

Reimbursements Using Conversion Factors

Setting a cost-based fee schedule is a critical step in the overall financial strategy of the practice, but there is another step that is just as important: negotiating third-party payer contracts that will cover the practice's expenses for the provision of contracted services. That type of coverage requires that the third-party payer's conversion factor for a service range must match or exceed the practice's blended cost per RVU for the same service range. For example, if the group's blended cost per RVU is $38.63, the conversion factor being negotiated with the third party must meet or beat that number. Otherwise, if the group accepts a conversion factor that is lower than its overall cost per RVU, it will lose money on each and every service provided to that plan's patients. If that

EXHIBIT 3.7. Fee Schedule Converted to a Factor of RBRVS

Health Care Clinic
Costs as a Factor of RBRVS
Six Month Period

	CPT	Mod	Cost/ Proc	Fee Schd	Factor	Freq.	Freq. Adj.
6	10040		64.12	67.06	0.96	2	1.91
7	10040	52	64.12	67.06	0.96	33	31.55
8	10060		61.49	63.51	0.97	40	38.73
163	54150		91.08	83.08	1.10	208	228.03
832	99440		218.74	194.89	1.12	65	72.95
833	99440	52	218.70	194.89	1.12	4	4.49
834				**Totals**		125,123	140,884.87
835			**RBRVS Factor**		1.13		
836							
837	**Note:**	Above codes represent a sample. ALL codes were included in					
838		final totals.					

contract is a major revenue source for the practice, it needs to be a profitable one, or the organization will begin a financial slide.

What if the carrier doesn't provide the practice with a conversion factor? What if it just provides the payment for each procedure? A conversion factor can easily be determined through the formulas provided in this text. Remember the formula for calculating the cost per procedure? The same principle can be used to calculate the conversion factor when the procedure fee is known. Apply simple algebra to solve for *x*, in this case the conversion factor.

$$\text{If} \ldots \text{RVU}_{total} * \text{Cost/RVU}_{blended} = \text{procedure cost, then} \ldots$$

$$\text{Procedure fee} \div \text{RVU}_{total} = \text{conversion factor}$$

$$\text{Example: } \$53.00 \div 1.37 = \$38.69$$

Cost Control versus Productivity

While increases or decreases in total costs can be determined simply by looking at the bottom line every period, wouldn't it be better to also know how the costs are changing relative to the business volume? The blended cost per RVU is an indication of a practice's cost control vs. its productivity (measured in RVUs). One could also examine the component cost per RVU to determine if it is increasing or decreasing relative to the volume of business.

For example, let's say that last year's total expenses for a fictional clinic were $1 million and the total RVUs were 40,000. The blended cost per RVU was therefore $25. This year the total expenses are 20 percent higher, but the productivity has increased only 5 percent. What does that do to the blended cost per RVU? It raises it to $28.57. Obviously, that's not the trend an administrator would want to continue, because it is costing more to run the operation this year than it did last year. What if the trend was reversed and productivity went up 20 percent (to 48,000 RVUs) while expenses rose 5 percent (to $1,050,000)? The result would be a blended cost per RVU of $21.88. That's good news! The practice is showing an improvement in cost efficiency over last year. In short, it gives the administrator a quick and easy way to determine the balance between expenses and productivity.

Another approach is to use total work RVUs for each CPT code to reflect volume (productivity). For this exercise you will need the CPT codes utilized (billed out for the time period being analyzed), frequency of billing per code, cost per procedure (using the formulas in this chapter) and reimbursement per procedure. This can be done per payer or for all payers combined. By sorting the data in descending order of volume, one can determine what codes comprise a certain volume of business. Monitoring the top volume codes over time allows the administrator to ferret out changes in coding patterns, treatment protocols and case mix. Fluctuation in the top volume coding mix can lead to changes in both revenues and expenses.

This exercise may also incorporate revenue instead of costs. Unless the practice's costs are way out of line with the associated reimbursements per procedure, the results should be nearly identical.

Note in Exhibit 3.8 that the top 20 codes account for 44.77 percent of the total costs, the top 27 codes account for more than 50 percent of the total costs, and 187 codes account for 80 percent of the total costs. Think about that. A mere 27 codes accounted for *half* of this orthopedic practice's volume! Why do an analysis that includes every single CPT code utilized within your practice when you can just pull out those codes that account for 80 percent of the total volume in terms of revenues or expense?

Key Cost per RVU Indicators

There are two key indicators that should be monitored every time a RVU cost analysis is performed: cost/RVU$_{blended}$ and cost/RVU$_{work}$. Why is the cost-per-work RVU a key indicator? If the practice were losing money, which of the three components, work, overhead or malpractice, would be the first on the chopping block to cut? It can't be malpractice since the medical practice has no control over professional liability premiums. With some minor exceptions, it probably won't be the overhead component because medical groups these days have ratcheted down the variable expenses as much as possible due to the decreased revenues associated with managed care. If the group is losing money, then, more

EXHIBIT 3.8. Orthopedic Practice Top Volume Codes

	A	B	C	D	E	K	L	M
	cpt	mod	description	freq	cost	total cost	volume	% total cost
2	99213		Office/outpatient visit, est	12,210	63.07	770140.9	6.01%	
3	99203		Office/outpatient visit, new	5,185	114.68	594596.1	4.64%	10.65%
4	27447		Total knee replacement	221	2,459.28	543499.9	4.24%	14.89%
5	99212		Office/outpatient visit, est	9,514	45.58	433618.6	3.38%	18.28%
6	99214		Office/outpatient visit, est	4,069	96.18	391354.8	3.05%	21.33%
7	99202		Office/outpatient visit, new	3,380	82.11	277539.6	2.17%	23.50%
8	20610		Drain/inject joint/bursa	3,265	83.74	273399	2.13%	25.63%
9	29881		Knee arthroscopy/surgery	290	909.94	263883.7	2.06%	27.69%
10	22612		Lumbar spine fusion	113	2,265.72	256026.4	2.00%	29.69%
11	63030		Low back disk surgery	182	1,381.09	251358.8	1.96%	31.65%
12	27130		Total hip replacement	107	2,314.47	247648.6	1.93%	33.58%
13	99204		Office/outpatient visit, new	1,277	167.94	214458.1	1.67%	35.26%
14	22554		Neck spine fusion	89	2,083.47	185428.6	1.45%	36.70%
15	29888		Knee arthroscopy/surgery	114	1,604.00	182855.7	1.43%	38.13%
16	27244		Repair of thigh fracture	95	1,770.78	168223.9	1.31%	39.44%
17	23420		Repair of shoulder	99	1,541.21	152579.6	1.19%	40.63%
18	99213	25	Office/outpatient visit, est	2,307	63.08	145514.9	1.14%	41.77%
19	72100		X-ray exam of lower spine	2,583	54.63	141120.9	1.10%	42.87%
20	99455		Disability examination	890	138.35	123128.7	0.96%	43.83%
21	63047		Removal of spinal lamina	71	1,696.32	120438.9	0.94%	44.77%
22	20550		Inj tendon/ligament/cyst	1,424	82.41	117356.3	0.92%	45.69%
23	27134		Revise hip joint replacement	35	3,242.77	113497	0.89%	46.57%
24	27236		Repair of thigh fracture	63	1,778.87	112068.6	0.87%	47.45%
25	29826		Shoulder arthroscopy/surgery	105	1,065.67	111895.7	0.87%	48.32%
26	69990		Microsurgery add-on	335	297.77	99751.31	0.78%	49.10%
27	99203	25	Office/outpatient visit, new	822	114.68	94264.66	0.74%	49.84%
28	73564		X-ray exam of knee, 4+	1,731	52.21	90372.05	0.71%	50.54%
188	25270		Repair forearm tendon/muscle	14	635.85	8901.963	0.07%	80.01%

than likely, the first place administration will look to cut costs is provider salaries and benefits. Now do you see why it is a key indicator? It is definitely a key indicator to those whom it affects!

That raises the question of how often a RVU cost analysis should be performed. This author recommends doing it on an annual basis, but no more than twice a year. If a cost analysis is performed more than once each year, an allowance must be made for year-end expenses and accruals. Because practice expenses (especially overhead) can vary considerably throughout the year, a monthly or quarterly RVU cost analysis can cause unnecessary anxiety. On the other hand, RVU productivity analysis can and should be performed at least quarterly, if not monthly. The trends in productivity can easily and frequently be tracked without the concerns of a cost analysis.

CONCLUSION

RVU cost analysis can be a powerful tool for medical practice management in today's competitive market. Cost analysis at the per (relative) unit level provides the administrator with a profitability analysis tool, cost-based fee schedules, contract negotiation with quantitative leverage, equitable provider compensation packages, etc. The two key cost per RVU indicators are the blended cost per RVU (used as the bottom line in managed care contract negotiation and to monitor the changes in cost relative to volume) and the cost per work RVU.

Note

1. Longhurst, P. (1991). Optimizing Physicians' Reimbursement Revenue, Part 1: Pricing Physicians' Services. Journal of Medical Practice Management 6(3):174–181.

CHAPTER **4**

RVUs in Managed Care Contracting

INTRODUCTION

In the "good old days" it was simple: Patients wanted to be healthy, and physicians wanted to be paid. Until the advent of managed care a few decades ago, if physicians weren't earning enough, they would simply raise their fees because the patients and/or their indemnity insurance plans would pay whatever rates were charged. In addition, today's patients not only want to be healthy; they also want to pay no more than a $10 copayment! Now, third-party payers tell the health care organization what they will allow or pay for services rendered, and few pay a practice's gross charges—unless gross charges are less than what the payer allows, or the provider has a monopoly in the market. On top of all that, physicians still want to be paid! Thankfully, after years of insurance plans ratcheting down the payment systems through capitation and of providers cutting back their services and operations to the point of bankruptcy, the pendulum is swinging back in some markets, and discounted fee-for-service is making a comeback. Just as Bob Dylan's song says "for the times, they are a-changin'."

RVUs can be used to track and analyze clinical productivity and costs, knowledge which in turn can be used as a tool when negotiating third-party payer contracts. Whether the discussion involves a discounted fee-for-service, a factor of RBRVS or a capitation contract, RVUs can provide information that is a distinct advantage at the bargaining table. Note the key words, "negotiating" and "bargaining." Before sitting down with an insurance carrier to sign on the bottom line, know the risks incurred with the acceptance of any contract, and vigorously negotiate the points that would be deal breakers. If you have the quantitative data to back up your analysis, you will have the justification for your position at the bargaining table. Use it wisely. The days when medical practices simply accepted third-party payer contracts just because they were offered are disappearing, except in some areas where the market leverage of the purchaser is overwhelming.

There are numerous reimbursement systems in the marketplace today, ranging from discounted fee-for-service (FFS) to capitation contracts and everything in between. Some contract types are fairly straightforward on a continuum of payer contract complexity. Easier contracts to understand and negotiate are those such as the discounted FFS or the managed care fee schedules. Others are more complicated, such as the ones that offer a factor of the RBRVS or a capitated contract. The discounted FFS is one of the simpler payer contracts because it is really just a percentage off the practice's own charges. Managed care fee schedules occur when the payer offers the practice a predetermined fee schedule for specific services. Contracts that offer a factor of the RBRVS are a bit more complicated because they involve conversion factors and RVUs, so they require a bit more understanding of the Medicare fee schedule and how it relates to a practice's own charges and costs. In a nutshell, if the Medicare fee for CPT 99213 is $50, and the contract offers a fee schedule that is 120 percent of Medicare, then the contract fee is $60. Therefore, the practice should see $60 allowed on explanation-of-benefit forms for that procedure for that contract year. Finally, on the opposite end of the complexity continuum from discounted FFS contracts are capitation contracts, an entirely new method of reimbursement for medical practices compared to discounted FFS contracts. Capitation contracts are discussed at the end of this chapter.

For more information on health care contracting in general, you may want to check out the *Health Care Contracting Desk Reference* published by Ingenix. It provides comprehensive information on contracting of all types, and includes valid industry data and models.

DISCUSSION

A Note on Fee Schedules

There are three main types of fee schedules: historical-based, market-based and cost-based.

Until recently, most ambulatory health care practices have based their charges per procedure on historical charges, on prevailing market rates and/or as a percentage of the Medicare physician payment schedule. When setting fees for the upcoming year, administrators using the historical method of determining fee schedules would typically review what their practices charged for procedures during the past year, and then maybe bump up the fees to what they believed the market should bear. That way they could adjust their fees to remain competitive regardless of whether the charges adequately covered practice expenses. In truth, this trend-based method of fee setting is arbitrary, subjective and potentially financially harmful. This historical-based fee schedule may not actually cover the cost of doing business, therefore it is not financially viable for medical practices in today's competitive markets.

A market-based fee schedule is based primarily on what the group thinks the market will bear based on the market research it has conducted or on what the managed care contracts are paying. Some administrators believe that a managed care contract matches what the market will bear. That is not usually the case. Do your homework before accepting any fee schedule as market driven.

It is best to use a cost-based fee schedule discussed in chapter 3. Calculate the cost per procedure based on RVU utilization and all direct and indirect expenses, then add a profit margin. By having a cost-based fee schedule, an administrator has a much greater knowledge of which managed care contracts the group can afford to accept. If the fee schedule is not cost-based (it is historical-based or market-based), then the practice runs the danger of not knowing whether or not a particular contract will be profitable, financially disastrous or somewhere in between. A medical practice that does not both set a cost-based fee schedule and work to ensure that the revenue generated covers costs will not remain financially viable.

DISCOUNTED FEE-FOR-SERVICE

Exhibit 4.1 displays a cost-based fee schedule for frequently used E&M codes for a hypothetical group practice. (If you need a refresher on cost-based fee schedules, you may want to revisit Chapter 3.) This is the group's normal fee schedule based on what it costs the physicians and nonphysician providers to provide E&M services and procedures to their patients. Only the top 20 codes (in terms of volume) are used for this example since it follows the standard 80/20 rule of business (80 percent of the volume is contained within the top 20 volume codes). This example shows the top 20 volume CPT codes in ascending order along with a brief description, the frequency each code has been utilized by all patients within the practice over the last year, the standard fee charged per procedure prior to any adjustments, and the total gross charges.

The basic concept for discounted fee-for-service managed care contracts is simple: Managed care organizations (MCOs) offer percentage rates or reimbursement for procedures and services that are a discount off of the medical practice's usual fee schedule. For example, the MCO contract might offer to reimburse at a rate of 80 percent of the group's current fee schedule. Another contract might pay the lesser of the group's fee or the contracted rate, so naturally groups make sure their fees are equal to or greater than the contract rate. This type of managed care contract can work well for those groups that negotiate reimbursements that cover their costs plus provide some margin for profit. On the other hand, if a practice's fee schedules are not based on the actual costs of providing services, the administrator will have no idea whether or not he or she can afford to accept the contract. After all, if you don't know your costs, how can you make sure your costs are covered by a managed care contract?

Exhibit 4.2 gives an example of a discounted FFS contract using the same CPT codes as in the previous exhibit. Now the CPT codes are sorted by volume. This discounted contract is offering a rate that is 85 percent of the group's regular fee schedule; thus it offers a 15 percent discount.

This type of contract arrangement was a good deal, while it lasted, for smart administrators who would simply increase their

EXHIBIT 4.1. Cost-based Fee Schedule for E&M Codes

	A	B	C	D	E
1	**E&M Fee Schedule**				
2					
3	**CPT code**	**Description**	**Frequency**	**Fee**	**Total Gross Charges**
4	99202	Office/outpatient visit, new	4365	$82	$357,930
5	99203	Office/outpatient visit, new	7121	$122	$868,762
6	99204	Office/outpatient visit, new	2341	$172	$402,652
7	99212	Office/outpatient visit, est	41,295	$50	$2,064,750
8	99213	Office/outpatient visit, est	105,374	$75	$7,903,050
9	99214	Office/outpatient visit, est	27,395	$110	$3,013,450
10	99215	Office/outpatient visit, est	2572	$150	$385,800
11	99222	Initial hospital care	1089	$195	$212,355
12	99223	Initial hospital care	2780	$245	$681,100
13	99232	Subsequent hospital care	6152	$105	$645,960
14	99233	Subsequent hospital care	2432	$155	$376,960
15	99238	Hospital discharge day	2286	$135	$308,610
16	99243	Office consultation	4065	$180	$731,700
17	99391	Prev visit, est, infant	4821	$110	$530,310
18	99392	Prev visit, est, age 1-4	3903	$125	$487,875
19	99393	Prev visit, est, age 5-11	2525	$120	$303,000
20	99394	Prev visit, est, age 12-17	2726	$140	$381,640
21	99395	Prev visit, est, age 18-39	4395	$143	$628,485
22	99396	Prev visit, est, age 40-64	7726	$165	$1,274,790
23	99397	Prev visit, est, 65 & over	2029	$195	$395,655

EXHIBIT 4.2. Discounted Fee-for-Service Contract Analysis

	A	B	C	D	E	F	G
1	E&M Discounted Fee-for-Service for MCO Contract						
2	85% of fee schedule (15% discount)						
3	CPT code	Description	Frequency	Fee	Total Gross Charges	85% of Fee	MCO Reimbursement
4	99213	Office/outpatient visit, est	105,374	$75	$7,903,050	$63.75	$6,717,592.50
5	99212	Office/outpatient visit, est	41,295	$50	$2,064,750	$42.50	$1,755,037.50
6	99214	Office/outpatient visit, est	27,395	$110	$3,013,450	$93.50	$2,561,432.50
7	99396	Prev visit, est, age 40-64	7726	$165	$1,274,790	$140.25	$1,083,571.50
8	99203	Office/outpatient visit, new	7121	$122	$868,762	$103.70	$738,447.70
9	99232	Subsequent hospital care	6152	$105	$645,960	$89.25	$549,066.00
10	99391	Prev visit, est, infant	4821	$110	$530,310	$93.50	$450,763.50
11	99395	Prev visit, est, age 18-39	4395	$143	$628,485	$121.55	$534,212.25
12	99202	Office/outpatient visit, new	4365	$82	$357,930	$69.70	$304,240.50
13	99243	Office consultation	4065	$180	$731,700	$153.00	$621,945.00
14	99392	Prev visit, est, age 1-4	3903	$125	$487,875	$106.25	$414,693.75
15	99223	Initial hospital care	2780	$245	$681,100	$208.25	$578,935.00
16	99394	Prev visit, est, age 12-17	2726	$140	$381,640	$119.00	$324,394.00
17	99215	Office/outpatient visit, est	2572	$150	$385,800	$127.50	$327,930.00
18	99393	Prev visit, est, age 5-11	2525	$120	$303,000	$102.00	$257,550.00
19	99233	Subsequent hospital care	2432	$155	$376,960	$131.75	$320,416.00
20	99204	Office/outpatient visit, new	2341	$172	$402,652	$146.20	$342,254.20
21	99238	Hospital discharge day	2286	$135	$308,610	$114.75	$262,318.50
22	99397	Prev visit, est, 65 & over	2029	$195	$395,655	$165.75	$336,306.75
23	99222	Initial hospital care	1089	$195	$212,355	$165.75	$180,501.75
24		Total			$21,954,834		$18,661,608.90
25		$ Variance				-$3,293,225.10	
26		% Variance				0.85	

fees. When the MCO offered to pay a percentage of the group's normal rate, the group wouldn't really be giving up any margin! MCOs soon discovered there was no way to control the medical practice's fees, so they started offering their own fee schedules to the practices.

MANAGED CARE FEE SCHEDULES

It didn't take long for MCOs to graduate from discounted FFS contracts to their own managed care fee schedules. There are a number of different ways to conduct an analysis of various payers' fee schedules. This text touches on only a few of the more common examples. Keep in mind that each health care market can be different in terms of what the third-party payers are offering.

Fee Schedule Comparisons

You could begin by comparing the medical practice's fee schedule to the discount offered or to the payer's fee schedule. This works well if the practice's fee schedule is cost-based and has sufficient profit built into it. It does not work as well if the fee schedule is not cost-based because the administrator will not be able to tell if the third-party payer's reimbursement will cover the cost of providing the service. Market-based fee schedules (those based on what practice administrators believe the market will bear and on the market research they have conducted) should not be used when negotiating managed care contracts because those fee schedules are not cost-based and, therefore, could potentially hurt the practice financially. The same rationale applies to historical-based fee schedules.

You may recall the discussion on cost-based fee schedules from chapter 3; if not, you will want to review it because it is critical to understand your own practice's costs and to know how to calculate a cost-based fee schedule before you begin any contract negotiations. It involves calculating the cost per procedure using the methodology detailed in chapter 3 to determine the break-even point for each procedure, then adding a profit margin to the bottom line.

Exhibit 4.3 provides a template for analyzing this type of managed care contract where contractors offer their own fee schedules. Although only the top 20 in volume of E&M codes are included in the example, you should perform a similar analysis on all CPT codes covered by the contract. For many groups, E&M codes represent the majority of the practice's work, so E&M codes are often included in examples and analyses. For this template you will need the CPT codes with modifiers (if applicable) and descriptions (columns A and B); the frequency of utilization per code (column C); the practice's gross (unadjusted) fee for each procedure (column D); and the MCO's proposed reimbursement per procedure (column F).

When you do a complete analysis on all CPT codes, it is highly recommended that you break the codes into ranges such as E&M, medicine, surgery, etc. since payers may reimburse at different rates depending on code category. In this example, all the practice's patients were included; the example assumes that the entire patient population within this group is comparable to the payer's patient population. If the contract were to cover patients of only specific age ranges, such as pediatric or geriatric, or only females, as in OB/GYN practices, then the patients included in the following analysis should be filtered to include only those who fit the profile. If the MCO shares the utilization data for its plan members included in the proposed question, then you may consider using that data instead. But if the service mix is very similar to your current patient population in terms of age, gender and general health, then your data will be as good, if not better, to use.

Once you have the data elements loaded into a spreadsheet, you will need to multiply the frequency (column C) by the medical practice's gross fee per procedure (column D) to get the volume-adjusted gross charges (column E). Then multiply the frequency (column C) by the MCO's proposed fee-schedule reimbursement (column F) to derive the volume-adjusted MCO reimbursement rate (column G). Subtract total gross charges (column E) from total reimbursement (column G) to derive the dollar variance (column H) between your gross unadjusted fees and the MCO's fee schedule. Finally, divide column G by column E to arrive at the percentage variance (or discount percentage) in column I. As you can see by both the total dollar variance and the

EXHIBIT 4.3. Managed Care Contract Analysis

MCO fee schedule for E&M codes

CPT code	Description	Frequency	Fee	Total Gross Charges	MCO Fee Schedule	MCO Total Reimbursement	$ Variance	% Variance
99213	Office/outpatient visit, est	105,374	$75	$7,903,050	$80.00	$8,429,920	526,870	106.67%
99212	Office/outpatient visit, est	41,295	$50	$2,064,750	$55.00	$2,271,225	206,475	110.00%
99214	Office/outpatient visit, est	27,395	$110	$3,013,450	$105.00	$2,876,475	(136,975)	95.45%
99396	Prev visit, est, age 40-64	7726	$165	$1,274,790	$160.00	$1,236,160	(38,630)	96.97%
99203	Office/outpatient visit, new	7121	$122	$868,762	$105.00	$747,705	(121,057)	86.07%
99232	Subsequent hospital care	6152	$105	$645,960	$95.00	$584,440	(61,520)	90.48%
99391	Prev visit, est, infant	4821	$110	$530,310	$110.00	$530,310	0	100.00%
99395	Prev visit, est, age 18-39	4395	$143	$628,485	$145.00	$637,275	8,790	101.40%
99202	Office/outpatient visit, new	4365	$82	$357,930	$75.00	$327,375	(30,555)	91.46%
99243	Office consultation	4065	$180	$731,700	$180.00	$731,700	0	100.00%
99392	Prev visit, est, age 1-4	3903	$125	$487,875	$115.00	$448,845	(39,030)	92.00%
99223	Initial hospital care	2780	$245	$681,100	$235.00	$653,300	(27,800)	95.92%
99394	Prev visit, est, age 12-17	2726	$140	$381,640	$135.00	$368,010	(13,630)	96.43%
99215	Office/outpatient visit, est	2572	$150	$385,800	$145.00	$372,940	(12,860)	96.67%
99393	Prev visit, est, age 5-11	2525	$120	$303,000	$125.00	$315,625	12,625	104.17%
99233	Subsequent hospital care	2432	$155	$376,960	$160.00	$389,120	12,160	103.23%
99204	Office/outpatient visit, new	2341	$172	$402,652	$140.00	$327,740	(74,912)	81.40%
99238	Hospital discharge day	2286	$135	$308,610	$125.00	$285,750	(22,860)	92.59%
99397	Prev visit, est, 65 & over	2029	$195	$395,655	$175.00	$355,075	(40,580)	89.74%
99222	Initial hospital care	1089	$195	$212,355	$195.00	$212,355	0	100.00%
Total				**$21,954,834**		**$22,101,345**	**146,511**	
					$ Variance		146,511	
					% Variance			1.00667291

total percentage variance, this is a good contract for this particular group because overall the group will earn additional revenue even though some codes lose money.

Fee Schedule Discounts

Some MCOs may offer discounted fee schedules that can be analyzed in a different manner. Exhibit 4.4 uses a different data set from the previous example to show you another method of analysis. Although only a few E&M codes are displayed in the example, all CPT codes covered by the contract are included in the totals at the bottom of the exhibit. As in the previous example, for this template you will need the CPT codes with modifiers and descriptions (columns A to C), preferably broken into CPT code ranges like E&M, medicine, surgery, etc.; the frequency of utilization per code (column F); the practice's gross fee or charge for each procedure (column E); and the MCO's proposed reimbursement per procedure (column D).

Once the spreadsheet is set up with the appropriate columns, start by multiplying the frequency (column F) by the medical practice's gross fee per procedure (column E) to get the volume-adjusted gross charges (column H). Next multiply frequency (column F) by the MCO's proposed reimbursement rate (column D) to derive the volume-adjusted MCO rate (column G). Finally, divide column G by column H to get the discount.

For example, look at the figures for CPT 90701 on line 34. Divide 28,353.16 by 35,278.75, for a factor of 0.8037. (You may want to round the number; it is up to you as the individual conducting the analysis.) That means that 80.37 percent of the gross charges for CPT 90701 are covered by the proposed contract, which in turn means that the proposed discount (column I) is 19.63 percent (calculated by subtracting 80.37 from 100) for that code. The sum of the adjusted MCO rates (column total G) divided by the sum of the adjusted gross charges (column total H) results in a factor of 78.95 percent for the E&M codes. Translation: 78.95 percent of gross charges are covered for E&M. The effective discount, then, is 100 percent minus 78.95 percent, or 21.05 percent.

When analyzing a managed care fee schedule contract, it is usually more important to look at the overall discount (weighted

EXHIBIT 4.4. Managed Care Fee Schedule Analysis

Fee Schedule Analysis – Compared to Gross Charges
MCO = *COST BENCHMARK*

CPT Code	mod	Description	MCO Reimbursement	Gross Charge	Freq (all pts)	MCO Reimb * Count	Gross Charge * Count	CPT Fee Discount	$ Variance
		EVAL & MGMT CODES							
90701		Dtp vaccine, im	17.45	21.71	1,625	28,353.16	35,278.75	-19.63%	($6,925.59)
90707		Mmr vaccine, sc	34.95	43.49	1,016	35,505.14	44,185.84	-19.65%	($8,680.70)
90737		Influenza B immunization	18.79	23.38	1,350	25,365.56	31,563.00	-19.64%	($6,197.45)
93000		Electrocardiogram, complete	32.86	50.33	704	23,134.07	35,432.32	-34.71%	($12,298.25)
96910		Photochemotherapy with UV-B	25.30	32.88	1,006	25,452.20	33,077.28	-23.05%	($7,625.08)
99050		Medical services after hrs	39.59	50.26	742	29,373.33	37,292.92	-21.24%	($7,919.59)
99070		Special supplies	29.64	26.93	1,243	36,843.02	33,473.99	10.06%	$3,369.03
99201		Office/outpatient visit, new	30.88	44.11	1,044	32,235.48	46,050.84	-30.00%	($13,815.36)
99203	52	Office/outpatient visit, new	66.50	79.76	516	34,314.05	41,156.16	-16.62%	($6,842.11)
99204		Office/outpatient visit, new	99.56	112.50	521	51,868.31	58,612.50	-11.51%	($6,744.19)
99211		Office/outpatient visit, est	14.92	21.24	3,425	51,117.10	72,747.00	-29.73%	($21,629.90)
99212		Office/outpatient visit, est	26.60	33.88	23,365	621,420.21	791,606.20	-21.50%	($170,185.99)
99213		Office/outpatient visit, est	37.77	53.89	5,327	201,175.75	287,072.03	-29.92%	($85,896.28)
99213	52	Office/outpatient visit, est	37.77	42.03	665	25,113.92	27,949.95	-10.15%	($2,836.03)
99214		Office/outpatient visit, est	57.96	91.15	1,175	68,106.41	107,101.25	-36.41%	($38,994.84)
99222		Initial hospital care	115.94	173.48	281	32,578.41	48,747.88	-33.17%	($16,169.47)
99231		Subsequent hospital care	36.30	45.66	624	22,649.52	28,491.84	-20.51%	($5,842.32)
99232		Subsequent hospital care	53.12	55.29	585	31,073.97	32,344.65	-3.93%	($1,270.68)
99291		Critical care, first hour	200.67	39.70	217	43,544.87	8,614.90	405.46%	$34,929.97
99391		Preventive visit, est,infant	28.50	35.53	1,264	36,020.97	44,909.92	-19.79%	($8,888.95)
99392		Preventive visit,est,age 1-4	30.89	38.36	1,110	34,292.01	42,579.60	-19.46%	($8,287.59)
99393		Preventive visit,est,age5-11	39.30	48.95	660	25,938.86	32,307.00	-19.71%	($6,368.14)
99431		Initial care, normal newborn	115.91	144.25	387	44,857.83	55,824.75	-19.65%	($10,966.92)
		% of Gross Charge Covered				1,560,334.14	1,976,420.57	78.95%	($416,086.43)
								-21.05%	
		TOTALS FOR ALL CODES				3,166,990.27	3,776,970.32	83.85%	
		% of Gross Charge Covered						-16.15%	

average) rather than at a particular procedure or service. As you will note in Exhibit 4.4, each line item has a different discount associated with it, but the overall discount for the E&M codes is 21.05 percent, and the discount for the entire range of codes (all categories and types) in the contract is 16.15 percent discount.

It is not that unusual for contracts to offer rates and discounts that vary with the type of procedure or service. Some services will have a deeper discount than others, so consider the volume of each of the deeply discounted line items. If the higher reimbursements are for procedures that are not routinely performed and the deeply discounted rates are for high volume procedures, then some renegotiation may be in order. For example, the MCO is offering a 34.71 percent discount on CPT 93000 (complete electrocardiogram), which may be acceptable since only 704 of those procedures were billed by this particular practice over the past year. However, the discount offered for CPT 99214, a high volume office visit code for an established patient, is 36.41 percent. It may be worth negotiating a higher reimbursement rate for that particular code. Overall, if the practice's fee schedule is cost-based and has enough buffer in it to absorb a 21 percent discount for the E&M codes in general and/or a 16 percent discount for all procedures and services, then this contract may be acceptable.

Conversion Factor Calculation

If the MCO offers a conversion factor (or multiple conversion factors, each one for a different range of services or procedures) rather than an entire fee schedule, the administrator needs to ensure that the conversion factor is higher than the medical practice's break-even point. That break-even point is the blended cost per RVU discussed in chapter 3 on costs. It is the point at which revenues match expenses, so there is neither gain nor loss. If the blended cost per RVU for the group is $40, then the proffered conversion factor needs to be at least $40, or the practice will lose money on every procedure billed to that particular MCO.

Conversely, if the managed care contract offers a fee schedule and doesn't give a conversion factor for a group of services, it is easy to calculate the conversion factor. The basic formula for pricing a procedure is:

$$RVU_{total} * \text{Conversion Factor} = \text{Procedure Reimbursement}$$

If you know what the total RVUs and the reimbursement are for a given procedure then simply divide the total RVUs into the reimbursement amount to obtain the conversion factor.

When the administrator has data about the actual cost of providing each service or procedure, he or she is much more likely to gain leverage in the contract negotiation process. A contractor who wants to do business will be more apt to be flexible in the reimbursement rates knowing that the administrator has the facts to back up the demands.

Conversion Factor of RBRVS

According to the American Association of Health Plans' 1998 annual report, more than half (56.3 percent) of the Health Maintenance Organizations (HMOs) paying fee-for-service to primary care physicians and to specialists base their fees on the Medicare fee schedule (the RBRVS) or a factor of it.[1] In other words, the majority of managed care contracts use a factor of the RBRVS (called a conversion factor [CF]) of Medicare, meaning that the rates are above or below Medicare's rates by some set amount. For example, a contract may be 140 percent (a factor of 1.40) or 85 percent (a factor of 0.85) of Medicare's standard reimbursement. If this is the case with your contract, then you will want to calculate your costs as a factor of the RBRVS so that an equitable comparison of your practice's costs and the managed care plan's rates can be made.

The other critical point to remember when negotiating a managed care contract based on a factor of the RBRVS is to ask the payer which year's Medicare fee schedule—both the conversion factor and the RVUs—it is using. It can make a significant difference in your analysis if you are using one year's fee schedule while the payer is using another year since the CF changes annually with the RBRVS. A CF is simply the number or factor by which RVUs are multiplied in order to calculate a reimbursement for a procedure. Expressed as a monetary figure, the CF converts RVUs into dollars.

FEE SCHEDULE CALCULATIONS
Geographic Practice Cost Indices

Most carriers use multiple or various conversion factors to adjust market conditions for the variance in reimbursement rates in locations across the nation. Just to add a little more complexity to the reimbursement scenarios, some carriers may use geographic adjustment factors (GAFs) for specific codes, rather than for all codes, or they may use a nominal factor multiplied by a CF. (Medicare's GAFs are called geographic practice cost indices or GPCIs as discussed below.) Insurance carriers that do not incorporate GAFs into the fee schedules might simply multiply the total RVUs by a CF as shown in Exhibit 4.5.

EXHIBIT 4.5. Fee Schedule Calculation without GAFs

	Work	Practice Expense	Malpractice	Total

CPT code 99213:
$(RVU_w = 0.67) + (RVU_{pe} = 0.69) + (RVU_m = 0.03) = 1.39$

Fee schedule calculations:

$(RVU_w + RVU_{pe} + RVU_m) * CF = Reimbursement$

$1.39 * 36.1992 = \$50.32$

Sometimes carriers pay a factor of the RBRVS when reimbursing physicians. For example, a carrier that pays 110 percent of Medicare may calculate the reimbursement for CPT code 99213 with a total RVU of 1.39 (prior to any GPCI adjustment) as follows:

$$1.39 * 36.1992 * 1.10 = \$54.35$$

If a carrier is competing in Colorado and basing fees on the RBRVS, it may offer less than 100 percent of the RBRVS since Medicare pays less in Colorado than in some other states. For example, a carrier paying RBRVS may initially calculate its fee to match Medicare's average GPCI-adjusted payment for that location (let's say, for example, it is 0.98) for 99213 as follows:

$$1.39 * 36.1992 * 0.98 = \$49.31$$

Medicare Fee Schedule Calculation

Medicare uses one CF for the entire United States instead of numerous conversion factors based on geographic location and market dynamics as used by other payers. In Exhibit 4.6 the conversion factor for calendar year 2002 is $36.1992. Recognizing that operating costs vary with location, CMS created geographic practice cost indices (GPCIs) to adjust individual codes for those differences. For example, it generally costs more to operate a clinic in urban New York City or Los Angeles than it does a similar clinic in rural North Dakota. GPCI adjustments, unique to the Medicare payment system, allow for the variance in expenses so that each practice is equitably reimbursed.

GPCIs, which have the same three components as the RVUs in the RBRVS, are typically updated on an annual basis. Both the GPCIs and the RBRVS are published by CMS annually in an issue of the *Federal Register,* usually available in early November for the following calendar year. To calculate a Medicare physician's fee schedule, as shown in Exhibit 4.6, each RVU component for a given CPT code is first multiplied by its corresponding GPCI. The three components are then summed, and this total is multiplied by the Medicare CF. This example shows the reimbursement that a nonfacility (such as an ambulatory care facility) in Colorado would receive from Medicare for office visit code 99213 in the year 2002.

CMS has assigned the state of Colorado GPCI values of less than 1.0, indicating that it is slightly less expensive to operate a practice in Colorado than in some other parts of the United States, such as Alaska or Rhode Island.

Comparing Charges and Costs to Fee Schedules

Your Charges in Relation to Medicare's Fees

As a practice administrator, it is nice to know your weighted average charge as a multiplier of Medicare (a figure that comes in very handy for many managed care contracts!). Exhibit 4.7 is an example to help determine your practice's fee schedule as a percentage of Medicare if you are not already establishing your fees as such. It builds on the example in Exhibit 4.1. As shown, this particular group practice's charges are approximately 149 percent of Medicare's fees using the 2002 conversion factor of $36.1992.

EXHIBIT 4.6. Medicare Fee Schedule Calculation Using GPCIs

	Work	Practice Expense	Malpractice	Total
CPT code 99213:	$RVU_w = 0.67$	$RVU_{pe} = 0.69$	$RVU_m = 0.03$	
Colorado GPCIs:	$GPCI_w = \underline{0.985}$	$GPCI_{pe} = \underline{0.992}$	$GPCI_m = \underline{0.840}$	
Adjusted RVUs:	0.65995	+ 0.68448	+ 0.0252	= 1.36963

Medicare's fee schedule calculations:

$$[(RVU_w * GPCI_w) + (RVU_{pe} * GPCI_{pe}) + (RVU_m * GPCI_m)] * CF = Reimbursement$$

$$1.36963 * 36.1992 = \$49.58$$

EXHIBIT 4.7. Fee Schedule as a Percentage of Medicare

	A	B	C	D	E	F	G
1	E&M Fee Schedule						
2							
3	**CPT code**	**Description**	**Frequency**	**Fee**	**Total Gross Charges**	**Total RVUs Per CPT**	**Frequency Adjusted RVUs**
4	99202	Office/outpatient visit, new	4365	$82	$357,930	1.7	7,420.50
5	99203	Office/outpatient visit, new	7121	$122	$868,762	2.54	18,087.34
6	99204	Office/outpatient visit, new	2341	$172	$402,652	3.61	8,451.01
7	99212	Office/outpatient visit, est	41,295	$50	$2,064,750	1	41,295.00
8	99213	Office/outpatient visit, est	105,374	$75	$7,903,050	1.39	146,469.86
9	99214	Office/outpatient visit, est	27,395	$110	$3,013,450	2.18	59,721.10
10	99215	Office/outpatient visit, est	2572	$150	$385,800	3.2	8,230.40
11	99222	Initial hospital care	1089	$195	$212,355	2.99	3,256.11
12	99223	Initial hospital care	2780	$245	$681,100	4.17	11,592.60
13	99232	Subsequent hospital care	6152	$105	$645,960	1.48	9,104.96
14	99233	Subsequent hospital care	2432	$155	$376,960	2.11	5,131.52
15	99238	Hospital discharge day	2286	$135	$308,610	1.83	4,183.38
16	99243	Office consultation	4065	$180	$731,700	3.2	13,008.00
17	99391	Prev visit, est, infant	4821	$110	$530,310	2.07	9,979.47
18	99392	Prev visit, est, age 1-4	3903	$125	$487,875	2.32	9,054.96
19	99393	Prev visit, est, age 5-11	2525	$120	$303,000	2.29	5,782.25
20	99394	Prev visit, est, age 12-17	2726	$140	$381,640	2.55	6,951.30
21	99395	Prev visit, est, age 18-39	4395	$143	$628,485	2.58	11,339.10
22	99396	Prev visit, est, age 40-64	7726	$165	$1,274,790	2.85	22,019.10
23	99397	Prev visit, est, 65 & over	2029	$195	$395,655	3.13	6,350.77
24					$21,954,834		407,428.73
25							
26	Gross charges/ Frequency Adjusted RVUs = Average weighted gross charge per RVU =						
27	$21,954,834/407,428.73 = $53.89						
28							
29	Average weighted gross charge per RVU/ Medicare CF = Average charge percent of Medicare =						
30	$53.89/$36.1992 = 1.49 or **149% of Medicare**						

Your Costs in Relation to Medicare's Conversion Factor

This section also applies to the discussion on cost analysis in chapter 3, but it appears here since we are discussing managed care contracts and the need for various types of contracts to cover practice expenses. The example in Exhibit 4.8 is a very practical and simple way to examine your practice costs, both individually and in total compared to the Medicare CF. Why use the Medicare figure? The majority of payers base their fees on the Medicare CF, so it is important to use the same standard unit of measurement when analyzing your costs and fees.

EXHIBIT 4.8. Practice Cost Analysis

		1999	2000	2001
Total Units of Service		698,284	740,181	829,002
Gross Charge/RVU		$68.02	$72.10	$80.75
Net Revenue/RVU		$44.00	$46.78	$53.26
Overhead Cost/RVU	−	$26.03	$28.43	$31.85
Operating Profit Margin	=	**$17.97**	**$18.35**	**$21.41**
Provider Cost/RVU	+	$18.46	$19.90	$20.98
Total Costs/RVU	=	**$36.73**	**$36.61**	**$38.26**
Medicare CF		$34.73	$36.61	$38.26
Costs as a Percentage of Medicare CF				
Gross Charge/RVU		195.85%	196.94%	211.06%
Net Revenue/RVU		126.69%	127.78%	139.21%
Overhead Cost/RVU	−	74.95%	77.66%	83.25%
Operating Profit Margin	=	**51.74%**	**50.12%**	**55.96%**
Provider Cost/RVU	+	53.15%	54.36%	54.84%
Total Costs/RVU	=	**104.89%**	**104.48%**	**110.79%**

You will note in Exhibit 4.8 that this analysis also includes a trend timeline, important because it allows you to see changes in your fees and charges in relation to the national standard, or Medicare.

Total units of service refer to total RVU volume for the practice. Calculating total RVUs based on clinical activity is discussed in chapter 2 on productivity. This example assumes that you know your total units of service. Using your practice's year-end financials, divide the gross charges, revenue and costs by the total RVU units to arrive at the dollar/RVU figures. It probably isn't important that all practice service charges and revenue have RVU values attached to them since we are only looking for ballpark guidelines to use.

As you can see by this particular example for 2001, the practice costs are 110.79 percent of the Medicare CF. This means that managed care contracts need to offer rates that are above the 110.79 percent break-even point in order for the group to make any profit. Determine the profit margin needed for your practice and negotiate for it.

Calculating Your Costs as a Factor of RBRVS

Exhibit 4.9 shows you how to calculate your practice's costs as a factor of the RBRVS. First, the cost per procedure must be calculated for each CPT code (with and without a modifier) billed out of the practice during the given time period. Typically, a full year of data are included in any analysis to provide the full range of service and procedure utilization figures. Next, divide each cost per procedure (column B) by the Medicare reimbursement (column C) for that procedure to derive a factor (column D). Multiply the factor (column D) by the CPT code utilization frequency (column E) to arrive at the frequency adjusted figure (column F), then total all the frequency adjusted numbers and divide by the sum of all the frequencies. The result is your practice's costs as a factor of the RBRVS.

Although the example in Exhibit 4.9 shows all codes combined together, you may want to categorize the codes according to E&M, medicine, surgery, etc. The factor will most likely differ for each code range because of the variance in types of procedures and the associated costs and reimbursements.

EXHIBIT 4.9. Practice Costs as a Factor of the RBRVS

A	B	C	D	E	F
CPT code	Cost/ Procedure	Medicare Reimbursement	Factor	Frequency	Frequency Adjusted
59400	$1,523.78	$1,380.83	1.10	389	429.27
59510-80	1,718.45	1,557.03	1.10	104	114.78
99212	26.27	23.54	1.12	23,365	26,074.70
All Other	X,XXX.XX	X,XXX.XX	X.XX	101,265	114,266.12
Totals				**125,123**	**140,884.87**
Cost Factor			**1.13**		

How do you then use this information during contract negotiations? Think of the factor as the bottom line or break-even point for your particular medical practice. Any figure below your bottom line will result in a consistent loss of revenue any time a plan member receives services because the plan pays less than your actual costs. In order for the contract to be profitable to your group, the proffered amount must be higher than your break-even point—in this case 1.13 or 113 percent of Medicare's rate. Just remember that, in this case, costs include physicians and non-physician providers.

Compare MCO FS to Medicare FS

Another way to use a factor analysis is to compare the MCO's fee schedule to the Medicare fee schedule. Exhibit 4.10 uses the same basic information from some of the previous managed care contract examples, but adds the Medicare fee schedule so that the MCO fee schedule as a factor of the RBRVS can be calculated.

There are two basic methods that can be used in this example. You could multiply the frequency (column C) by the MCO fee schedule (column F), then divide the result by the frequency (column C) multiplied by the Medicare fee schedule (column H), as follows:

$$\frac{\textbf{(Frequency * MCO Fee)} = (237,392 * 2,660) = 631,462,720}{\textbf{(Frequency * Medicare Fee)} = (237,392 * 1,781) = 422,557,760}$$

$$= 1.49$$

As you can see, the E&M factor of 1.49 calculated in this formula is a different result from that in Exhibit 4.10 because the denominators are different. Either method can be used, as long as it is used consistently to avoid confusion.

Another way to approach this calculation is suggested as follows by the chief financial officer of a large orthopedic group. To calculate the factor (column I) divide the MCO fee schedule (column F) by the Medicare fee schedule (column H). This gives you the factor per line item for each procedure. Then calculate the frequency-adjusted RVU factor by multiplying the factor by the frequency (column C). There are two ways to derive the overall or

EXHIBIT 4.10. Factor Analysis to Compare MCO and Medicare Fee Schedules

Factor of RBRVS for E&M codes

CPT code	Description	Frequency	Fee	Total Gross Charges	MCO Fee Schedule	Medicare Fee Schedule	RVU Factor	Frequency Adjusted RVU Factor
99213	Office/outpatient visit, est	105,374	$75	$7,903,050	$80	$50	1.59	167536.59
99212	Office/outpatient visit, est	41,295	$50	$2,064,750	$55	$36	1.52	62742.409
99214	Office/outpatient visit, est	27,395	$110	$3,013,450	$105	$79	1.33	36450.638
99396	Prev visit, est, age 40-64	7726	$165	$1,274,790	$160	$103	1.55	11982.042
99203	Office/outpatient visit, new	7121	$122	$868,762	$105	$92	1.14	8132.0042
99232	Subsequent hospital care	6152	$105	$645,960	$95	$54	1.77	10908.857
99391	Prev visit, est, infant	4821	$110	$530,310	$110	$75	1.47	7077.1842
99395	Prev visit, est, age 18-39	4395	$143	$628,485	$145	$93	1.55	6823.5158
99202	Office/outpatient visit, new	4365	$82	$357,930	$75	$62	1.22	5319.8283
99243	Office consultation	4065	$180	$731,700	$180	$116	1.55	6316.6106
99392	Prev visit, est, age 1-4	3903	$125	$487,875	$115	$84	1.37	5344.529
99223	Initial hospital care	2780	$245	$681,100	$235	$151	1.56	4327.9041
99394	Prev visit, est, age 12-17	2726	$140	$381,640	$135	$92	1.46	3986.7634
99215	Office/outpatient visit, est	2572	$150	$385,800	$145	$116	1.25	3219.5118
99393	Prev visit, est, age 5-11	2525	$120	$303,000	$125	$83	1.51	3807.4739
99233	Subsequent hospital care	2432	$155	$376,960	$160	$76	2.09	5094.5066
99204	Office/outpatient visit, new	2341	$172	$402,652	$140	$131	1.07	2507.9754
99238	Hospital discharge day	2286	$135	$308,610	$125	$66	1.89	4313.5633
99397	Prev visit, est, 65 & over	2029	$195	$335,655	$175	$113	1.54	3133.8398
99222	Initial hospital care	1089	$195	$212,355	$195	$108	1.80	1961.9699
Totals		237,392			$2,660	$1,781		360987.72

E&m Factor = 360,987.72 divided by 237,392 =   1.52

blended factor. You could calculate the average of the factors in column I by summing them and dividing by the number of factors (20 in this case). That would give you a factor of 1.5125. You can also divide the sum of the frequency-adjusted factors (column J) by the frequency (column C), as in Exhibit 4.10. The result of 1.52 is slightly different in this calculation because of rounding.

As you can see, there is more than one way to perform a factor analysis. These examples have been provided only to encourage you to think about how to use various methodologies when calculating your practice costs and comparing them to third-party payer rates.

CAPITATION CONTRACTS

RVUs may also be used to calculate or substantiate or negotiate per-member per-month (PMPM) capitation rates. Capitated contracts can be quite complicated, covering either specific service ranges or all medical services within the health care organization; they also address utilization (frequency of use of those services). In addition, there are numerous types of capitated contracts that may include primary care only, a full professional "cap" contract including all specialties, or even a global cap contract that includes expenses for all facilities (both inpatient and outpatient). Keep in mind, too, that age, gender, copayments and benefits may make a difference in the cap rates for a particular contract.

DISCUSSION
A Note about Copayments

Although mentioned earlier in this chapter, copayments are commonly used in contexts other than capitated contracts. Even if a copayment is only $10 or $20, the operational and financial impact of copayments is not trivial. For instance, let's say you have a Level 2 established patient office visit, and your contract rate for that service will be $30. If that particular plan has a $20 copayment, the insurance company will only pay the practice $10. If you don't collect the copayment, you lose the $20. Can you see the cumulative financial impact of copayments, deductibles or percentages within the plan? You have to know some of the operational issues in the contract, or your practice may be in for a rough financial ride throughout the length of the contract.

Your front office staff *must* collect the copayments at the time services are rendered. If the practice must bill the patient for the copayment, the cost of processing the bill and collecting the payment will eat up about $8 out of a $10 copayment.

Negotiating Capitation Contracts

Capitated contracts are concerned with utilization of services and assumption for the risk of providing patient care under a predetermined payment arrangement. In theory, the focus is on preventive services and health maintenance. It is much less expensive to prevent disease or to treat it in its early stages, rather than waiting until the patient is in the grasp of a full-blown expensive disease that will be very costly to all parties. The managed care plan will pay a predetermined amount per covered plan member per month. The practice will receive those monies regardless of whether or not the member visits the clinic or utilizes any services—but the practice also assumes the risk associated with those patients who contract a serious or even catastrophic illness. (That's what stop loss insurance covers, and why it is critical to have it when the practice has at-risk managed care contracts for services not directly controlled by the practice!) The result is that the fewer patients seen within the practice, the more money the practice makes. More patients seen in the office mean less profit. Obviously, this is a complete reversal of the old fee-for-service market dynamics. Think of it in terms of this simple equation:

(Number of plan members * capitation rate) – expenditures = profit

Plugging various numbers into each of the parts of the equation will give you an overall feel for how capitated contracts affect the revenue and, consequently, the profit. To give you a feel as to how this equation works, let's play out a few scenarios:

Scenario 1

(1,000 members * $50 cap rate PMPM) – $25,000 expenditures = $25,000 profit

Scenario 2

(1,000 members * $25 cap rate PMPM) – $25,000 expenditures = break-even point

Scenario 3

(1,000 members * $20 cap rate PMPM) – $25,000 expenditures = ($5,000) loss

This type of quick-and-dirty analysis will give you some idea on how the profit-and-loss scenarios would work in a capitated environment, but it is really much more complicated than it appears. There are so many different options within capitated contracts that it is impossible to provide a comprehensive guide to negotiating all of them in this chapter.

The insurance carrier maintains extensive actuarial data, including utilization of services, on patient populations such as those included in the contract under negotiation. Even though the carrier may not have utilization data on any one specific organization, rest assured that it has estimated its utilization based on millions of data points from similar populations. Not having utilization data for the group's own patient population means that the practice administrator loses a great deal of leverage in the negotiations. After all, if a practice's utilization and cost of services is not known, how can one negotiate with a carrier to cover those costs?

The point to remember is not to enter into any contract negotiation without prior knowledge of what the organization can afford to accept that will cover its costs associated with the volume and types of procedures covered under the managed care plan. Also be sure to closely consider safeguards such as stop loss insurance, floor and ceiling provisions, etc. This chapter on contract types is merely an overview; because capitation contracts in particular by nature are very complicated, readers are advised to exercise extreme caution and consult experts prior to signing on the dotted line. Consider that among the many complexities in managed care contracting there are both upside and downside risks, bonus and incentive plans, withholds, breakouts by specialty, etc.

Key Negotiation Points

There are overall a few key points to remember when negotiating a capitated contract. First, try to keep high-volume, costly, routine procedures that you can't control (such as immunizations) out of the contract. Immunizations are mandated by federal and state law, so there is no discretion on whether to provide these types of services and procedures. Furthermore, you have no control over the cost of immunizations. If you have no discretion or flexibility in the provision of services, then you also have no control over the costs associated with those types of services. In such situations, try to negotiate a fee-for-service rate instead of a cap rate to ensure that your costs are at least covered. Review the contract carefully to see what ICD-9 and CPT codes are included and excluded in the coverage plan so that surprises are avoided once the contract is signed.

Second, be sure to "carve out" any procedures or services that your practice does not or cannot offer. For example, primary care practices would be wise to exclude specialty procedures, such as those performed by neurologists or cardiologists, since, obviously, a primary care practice would not perform brain or open-heart surgery—unless, of course, the practice is willing to accept full professional services risk.

Third, know some basic demographic details about your current patient mix (such as gender, age and overall health) and compare them to the patient mix covered in the managed care plan. If it is significantly different from that of your current patient population, you'll need to gather additional actuarial information on the proposed plan members to ensure that the needs of these plan members can be met through your practice.

Fourth, find out what procedures and services are most frequently utilized by the members of the managed care plan. Utilization data are available from both the insurance carrier and from an actuary. You may also want to check those statistics against state-based data, if available. Keep in mind that Medicaid and Medicare managed care contracts imply that you will be accepting federal and state government-funded programs. If that is the case, you will want to negotiate separate and generally higher rates to care for these higher-risk patients who typically require more care and have more visits. Logically, people in the last few years of their lives require more health care services for both acute and chronic conditions than at any other time of their life cycle. According to one expert in the field, you should negotiate for rates that are three to five times higher than commercial rates in order to ensure profitability.[2] While that may be a good rule of thumb, you should also examine it relative to current market conditions. Finally, analyze the data carefully before making any deals. Know if your practice will make or lose money before signing the dotted line, and be sure to negotiate a reasonable exit or termination provision for the contract, just in case.

Critical data elements include cost per RVU, cost per procedure, expected utilization (frequency) of each service category and the number of plan members in the contract. Typically, capitated contracts are based on service utilization per 1,000 people in the patient population, but sometimes contracts are based on service utilization per 10,000 people due to the rarity of some disease conditions. Actuarial data, available from either the insurance carrier or an actuary, provide more accuracy and a better benchmark, but an RVU methodology can be used as a reasonable alternative in most cases.

Calculating Capitation Rates

Exhibit 4.11 gives a simplified example of the PMPM formula using fictitious numbers for illustration purposes only. More realistic illustrations would also include age/gender bands found within the patient populations since those may dramatically affect the results of any analysis. To calculate a PMPM bottom-line capitation rate for each service category, complete the following steps:

For the first step, arrange the data elements in a spreadsheet program with columns for the CPT codes, utilization frequency of each of those codes, the cost per procedure and total cost per procedure. In the first column, input the CPT codes billed out by the practice during the past 12 months, and separate the codes into service ranges using the AMA's CPT categories as a guide. In the second column input the total utilization (frequency of billing) for each code during the same time period. This information is available from the practice's billing system. The reason for using a 12-month time period is that most third-party payer contracts are for 12 months. Utilization is often based on a per-member year.

EXHIBIT 4.11. Simplified PMPM Formula

CPT	1 year of Utilization	*	Cost / Procedure	= Total Cost
99201	100		$23.85	$2,385
99202	1,000		37.65	37,650
99203	500		51.71	25,855
99215	120		70.84	8,501
Others	780		Average	10,609
Total Costs				**$85,000**
Divide by	12,000 member months		=	**$7.08 PMPM**

Using the formulas previously discussed in chapter 3 on costs, plug the cost of each procedure into the third column. Next, multiply the utilization for each CPT code within a range of service by the cost per procedure to get a total cost for each code, then sum the total costs for each service range. The total cost figure is the numerator in the PMPM formula.

Multiply 12 (months) by the number of capitated plan members to derive the number of member months. This number will be the denominator. Divide the total costs for each of the service categories by the number of per-member months to arrive at the PMPM cost for the service range. Repeat these steps for each range of service and add all the PMPMs. Finally, divide the total costs by the total member months to get the PMPM cap rate, in this case $7.08. Some contracts may offer a PMPM rate for individual service ranges; others may offer one global PMPM figure to cover all services under contract. In this example, the contract covers 1,000 lives for a period of 12 months.

Exhibits 4.12 and 4.13 provide another method of calculating a cap contract's PMPM rate for a 12-month contract. For this hypothetical situation, let's assume that the contract is for 1,000

EXHIBIT 4.12. Units of Service Per Member Year

CPT	% of Total	Expected Utilization	Total RVU per CPT	Adjusted RVU Units
99202	10% of 3,200	= 320	1.70	544.0
99212	10% of 3,200	= 320	1.00	320.0
99203	30% of 3,200	= 960	2.54	2,438.4
99213	30% of 3,200	= 960	1.39	1,334.4
99204	10% of 3,200	= 320	3.61	1,155.2
99214	10% of 3,200	= 320	2.18	697.6
Totals:		**3,200**		**6,489.6 units**

adult members for primary care only. We know from various survey reports on primary care utilization that we can expect an average of 3.2 office visits per year per adult enrollee, for a total of 3,200 visits (1,000 members * 3.2 visits). The exhibit is divided up into Level 2 visits (CPT codes 99202 and 99212), Level 3 visits (CPT codes 99203 and 99213) and Level 4 visits (CPT codes 99204 and 99214), which includes both new and established patients. Utilization for these codes normally follows a bell-shaped curve, meaning that the Level 3 visits are the most commonly coded for primary care physicians. We'll assume for this example that the curve applies to our contract population.

As you can see in Exhibit 4.12, there are 6,489.6 units of service per member year. The next step is to calculate the group's contract target rate, which will cover the practice's costs of these procedures and services. For this exercise, we'll assume that the administrator has calculated the cost per RVU for the group to be $46 (that is 121.1 percent of Medicare), compared to the Medicare conversion factor of $38 and the group's average charge per RVU of $57 (that is $57/$38 or 150 percent of Medicare). This cost per RVU is the break-even point for any contract negotiation because to accept less would mean losing money every time one of the contract's enrollees visits the clinic. In order to turn a bit of a profit on the contract, however, the administrator sets a contract target rate of $47.50 (or 125 percent of Medicare). This is not a scientific calculation; the administrator knows his or her costs are 121.1 percent of Medicare and that the practice needs to cover its costs, so the contract target rate is set at 125 percent of Medicare.

Next, calculate the required funding for the contract, and then divide it by the total member months to derive the per-member per-month rate. The complete calculation is shown in Exhibit 4.13.

Sometimes the capitation contract requires the medical practice to charge a copayment for office visits. If that is the case, then the group can accept a lower PMPM because of the revenue that will be generated from the copayments. (This assumes that the front desk employees know that copayments are due at the time services are rendered and that they collect the copayment prior to the patient's departure that day.)

EXHIBIT 4.13. Calculation for PMPM Rate

**Contract Target Rate * Units per Member Year
= Required Funding for the Contract**

Calculation: $47.50 * 6,489.6

= $207,005

1,000 members * 12 months = 12,000 member months, so...

$207,005/12,000 = $17.25 PMPM

For example, let's say that a $10 copayment will be due at the time of the office visit. This amounts to total additional revenue of $32,000 ($10 * 3,200 visits). Using the previous example of $207,005 total revenue dollars, we would then subtract the $32,000 in copayment revenue to get a new total of revenue generated from the cap contract of $175,000. The final step would be to divide the $175,000 by the 12,000 member months to derive a PMPM rate of $14.58. See Exhibit 4.14 for the formula.

The important point to remember with copayments is that the money MUST be collected at the time the service is rendered. Front desk staff must not allow the patients to be seen if the copayment cannot be paid up front because the cost of follow-up collection efforts negates any benefit of charging the copayment. Incidentally, the theory behind copayments is that utilization will decrease when patients have to pay for an office visit. In reality, most group practices will probably say that is not the case, unless perhaps the copayment is $20 or more.

While capitated contracts make sense intuitively for a health care system that is attempting to control the rapid escalation in costs, the number of pure capitated contracts has declined since 2000. Historically, most groups were not organizationally ready, either managerially or structurally, for the financial shock of managing complex capitation arrangements with a preset amount of revenue, which led to serious financial trouble. In order to succeed under a capitated contract, the medical group must run an exceptionally tight ship and have cost-accounting capabilities. Medical groups in the 1990s simply weren't ready for that drastic of a change in revenue generation after decades of fee-for-service and discounted fee-for-service contracts. Many medical practices

---

EXHIBIT 4.14. PMPM Rate with Copayment Revenue

$207,005 contract revenue
– 32,000 copayment revenue
$175,000 new contract revenue

$175,000/12,000 member months = $14.58 PMPM

in California, widely considered a bellwether state for health care, were losing so much money that they had to close their doors due to poor utilization management and inadequate capitation dollars. It was a tough lesson to learn in health care economics, but it is hoped that better reimbursement mechanisms will result. Current trends are leaning towards hybrid or customized payment systems that include discounted FFS, RVUs and capitation for certain procedures. In addition, plans are giving bonuses for meeting certain quality indicators and utilization benchmarks.

CONCLUSION

No matter what type of managed care contract is offered to a medical group practice, RVUs can often provide the quantitative data analyses necessary to successfully negotiate a profitable agreement. As you have seen in this chapter, contracts can be very complicated. There are numerous types of managed care contracts and even more ways to analyze the contracts compared to your fee schedules. If you are new to managed care contracting, it is best to consult with an expert so that you can negotiate the best possible arrangement with the third-party payer.

Notes

1. Fitzgerald, P., CT. Maples. (1998). AAHP Annual Industry Survey, 1998. 1999 Industry Profile: A Health Plan Reference Book. pp. 96.
2. Miscowic, A., McCally, JF. (1996, January/February). Using RVUs and RBRVS to Improve Practice Management and Bottom Line Revenues. Group Practice Journal. pp. 34–40.

CHAPTER **5**

Provider Compensation Using RVUs

INTRODUCTION

In days gone by, physician compensation was simple. Having seniority and generating a lot of revenue meant more money in the physician's pocket. Productivity and revenue went hand in hand, so the compensation was determined by those two elements. Missing from the standard equation, however, was the utilization of services (efficiency), quality and outcomes of care (effectiveness), patient satisfaction, etc. If the physicians wanted to make more money, they would raise their rates and see more patients. Problem solved. In today's managed care environment of declining reimbursement, however, a physician must be efficient, effective and receive good grades from patient satisfaction surveys in order to benefit financially. Compensation formulas today include a variety of measures and incentives, but all basically aim to reward both individual and team productivity while simultaneously providing high quality and cost-efficient care. Any medical practice that pays its physicians based on productivity needs to first know whether or not each provider is covering his or her costs. RVUs can provide that information and more at the per-provider level.

The purpose of this chapter is not to provide a detailed cookbook on how to design and implement a compensation formula. There are many other resources (a few are listed at the end of this chapter) that cover this subject in detail. The balance of this chapter will be dedicated to how the reader might use relative values

in a compensation formula. We will focus on a production allocation model and an expense allocation model. The examples will
be fairly simplistic in order to demonstrate the methodology. In
fact, the reader is only limited by his or her imagination (or toler-
ance for complex mathematical models) in designing a compensation formula that incorporates numerous methodologies to various degrees. For instance, a formula could be based on allocation
of production by using RVUs and an allocation of expenses with
one-half split equally and the balance based on practice cost RVUs
associated with the individual production RVUs. At the end of the
chapter are two real-life examples of physician compensation systems to show you how diverse the plans can be in medical group
practice.

COMPENSATION CONSIDERATIONS

There are a wide variety of physician compensation methodologies, almost as many methodologies as there are medical groups.
Compensation plans should relate to the practice's goals, objectives,
values, culture, marketplace and the types of data available for
measurement. According to Susan Cejka and Lesley Coleman of
Cejka & Company, there are four primary types of compensation
plans:

1. Production for the fee-for-service (FFS) markets;

2. Salary plus incentive;

3. Capitation; and

4. A combination model which uses both FFS and capitation.[1]

More simply put, very few plans are exactly alike, but most fall
into distinct categories that seem to range from guaranteed
salaries to an equal division of the pie (money left over after paying all expenses) to a complex formula that rewards productivity
and/or collections, allocates expenses and offers a variety of bells
and whistles under the heading of incentives and bonuses.

Each model has its strengths and weaknesses that need to be
recognized and understood. A guaranteed salary is easily under-

stood and calculated. An equal division of the profits requires more complex accounting—which should be in place anyway—but more importantly, requires an essentially equal distribution of the workload in order to be sustainable. Significant variations (say 10 percent) must be accounted for by adjusting the compensation to avoid discord and pressure to change the plan, or worse, to replace the individual(s). Compensation based on productivity, collections, expenses, incentives, etc. greatly increases the complexity of calculation, but it also offers opportunities to provide rewards or penalties for certain behaviors. Productivity, expense management, team work, patient and provider satisfaction, health care costs, and quality are all examples of outcomes that might be influenced by a compensation formula. Since many compensation plans have both base salary and incentive or bonus components, it should be understood that there must be minimum standards, sometimes called performance levels or thresholds, that must be met in order to be eligible for the incentive. Beyond covering one's costs, these standards might include a minimum number of ambulatory and hospital encounters per week or a minimum number of new patients in a given time period, completion of medical records and billing documents within a specified time after services have been rendered or participation in marketing efforts and community service events.

It is also important to take into consideration other components of compensation since, in the aggregate, they amount to a significant sum of money. Retirement plan contributions (pensions, 401(k) and profit sharing), deferred compensation arrangements, insurance plans (disability, dental, health, life, etc.), vacation, and time off for continuing medical education (CME) are frequently referred to as benefits. However, it is often possible to distribute cash in lieu of a "benefit," so each group must decide how these various items will be treated with respect to their compensation plan. Some groups choose to treat these items as expenses to each physician, while others consider them to be part of the group overhead. Regardless of how the items are treated, it is important that they be recognized as components of compensation.

Expert advisors in the physician compensation field generally have certain guidelines and "rules" that should be followed when designing a formula. In general, bonuses or incentives for individual performance with additional profit-sharing opportunities for group performance are among the more effective in promoting the behaviors desired to meet the practice's goal and objectives. Following are a few of the more common axioms that apply to physician compensation formulas:

1. Adequate staff and information resources need to be available to support the formula. The more complex the formula, the more resources required. The KISS (keep it simple) principle works best here.

2. Make it as understandable as possible. It is hard for the physicians to support something that they don't understand; therefore, easy comprehension is critical to the plan's success.

3. Physician interaction in the development of a formula generally increases the probability of successful implementation and subsequent acceptance. People support what they help create. Get physician buy-in early and often. The process is as important as the product.

4. The formula should be equitable to the participants. If it isn't perceived to be fair, then, likewise, it would be considered to be equally unfair. There is no standard formula that fits all situations, and generally formulas already in place are being constantly changed to meet the needs of the medical group. If the formula does not promote good will and teamwork among the physicians and staff, it's time to reevaluate the plan. It also needs to reflect the practice's overall goals of high quality health care, good outcomes, and both patient and provider satisfaction.

5. Each physician within an organization must help to control costs and utilization in order for the entire practice to prosper. Keep this in mind when designing incentives and bonuses, and give physicians a financial stake in improving care and outcomes.[2]

6. And finally, it doesn't matter how you divide the pie if you don't have adequate pie (money) at the end of the day to meet expenses. Remember: No margin, no mission.

Small-Group Compensation Plans

There is no one-size-fits-all plan when it comes to pay systems in medical groups. When it comes to small groups, however, there are a few additional comments worth mentioning because of the impact each individual physician can have on the group as a whole.

A small group's administration may not have the time or resources to implement and monitor a complicated plan that involves multiple measurements of productivity and behavior. Small groups may not have the expensive, sophisticated practice management systems that the larger groups have, so staff may not have all the same data at their fingertips that their counterparts in the larger groups do. Just keep in mind that whatever behaviors are rewarded will be increased; so if an individual's "eat what you kill" behavior is paramount to a physician's pay, then teamwork suffers. However, if teamwork is at the top of the list, what is the incentive for an individual physician to perform at his/her best? Tricky, isn't it?

Physicians in small groups tend to take a more active role in the development and administration of their compensation plans. If even one physician in a small group leaves, the burden of responsibility and the stress on the income level of the others increases. In other words, since there are fewer physicians in a small group environment to share both the revenue and the responsibilities of patient care, every doctor has considerably more power to influence the decision and to veto anything they dislike. Therefore, the plan should be as simple as possible to administer and monitor, have the support and buy-in of all the physicians, and at the same time promote the values and goals of the practice. Plans that best fit the small group may include both an individual and team approach, but most importantly they need to make sure that the group is compliant with the self-referral law requirements (such as Stark regulations).[3]

Pros and Cons of Using RVUs in Physician Compensation

Pros

Production measurement tools should be payer neutral and objective, and they should not be linked to charges or collections. RBRVS RVUs are a proven, consistent and neutral method of measuring physician work across specialties; therefore, many multispecialty groups use RVUs in their pay systems. Work RVUs were designed to measure the amount of a physician's time, effort, skill and intensity that went into direct patient care. Physicians perceive RVUs as both logical and understandable. Unlike other productivity measures, RVUs can track differences in practice patterns, and they encourage cost-effective care. Because they are seen as both fair and effective, work RVUs are the most commonly used metric among large groups that use productivity data.[4]

RVUs are payer neutral, so any payer-mix discrimination is eliminated. What sets work RVUs apart from the rest of the field (clinical hours, patient encounters, collections and charges to name a few) is that they represent "a single scale that isolates and measures physician specific resource requirements for the full spectrum of codes."[5] Furthermore, RVUs are continually updated by a standing committee comprised of 30-plus specialties known as the RBRVS Update Committee (RUC). RVUs encourage a group-oriented practice approach, and link physician compensation to the services provided rather than to the quality of the patient's insurance coverage.[6]

Cons

On the other hand, CMS uses the RVU scale to determine physician payments; and when there are updates to the scale, they must be budget neutral so more codes are affected. This can have implications for tracking RVUs from year to year since changes can be caused by factors other than just fluctuations in productivity. Comparing one specialty to another is a challenge, and must be done carefully. For example, while it might be all right to compare a plastic surgeon to an otolaryngologist, it would be inappropriate to compare most surgical specialties to internists or family practitioners.

Bruce A. Johnson, JD, MBA, a principal of the MGMA Health Care Consulting Group, notes several potential problems with using RVUs in compensation plans.[7] Physicians who are familiar with the old adage of "more work equals more pay" may see RVUs as disconnecting the relationship between work and money. This could drive down productivity, which may or may not be a good thing: It can be good as long as it doesn't drive down quality of care, outcomes or patient satisfaction. Johnson also points out that there is little benchmarking data on RVUs in compensation plans, and those specialty-specific RVUs can lead to overly complex plans.

RVUs, which are subject to "gaming" like other productivity measurement tools, are still volume driven. (Gaming is an intentional inappropriate behavior designed to increase compensation.) When a provider discovers that higher coding can mean higher RVUs, upcoding may result, which in turn may bring about coding audits and severe penalties. Administrators must be careful that the plan does not provide an incentive for bad behaviors such as improper coding. Some of these cons can be overcome as physicians become more familiar with how RVUs work and as more benchmarking data become available. A little provider education may go a long way in making everyone more comfortable with incorporating RVUs into the payment system.

USING RVUS TO PAY FOR PRODUCTION

The American Medical Group Association's (AMGA) *2001 Medical Group Compensation & Productivity Survey* indicated a significant increase in the percentage of medical groups reporting the use of RVUs to measure physician productivity. The AMGA data are based on responses received from 220 multispecialty and single-specialty medical groups across the country representing some 27,000 physicians. The survey data reflected an increase in the use of RVUs from 8 percent of the groups in 1999 to 28 percent in 2000.[8]

According to the MGMA *Physician Compensation and Production Survey Reports* from 1997 through 2001, there is a slow, but steady upward trend from approximately 12 percent to 19 percent of respondents over those five years in the number of groups that include RVUs as part of their compensation methodology. Other productivity measures surveyed include gross charges, adjusted charges, collections, patient encounters and patient panel size. Interestingly, the use of collections has shown a downward trend over that same time period from approximately 66 percent in the 1997 report to 49 percent of respondents in the 2001 report. During the second half of the 1990s, the RBRVS was undergoing major renovations to the calculations of each of the components from charge-based values to resource-based values. Now that all three components are resource based, there should be only minor tweaking of some of the values each year. Time will tell whether this may have settled the jitters that made practice administrators shy away from using RVUs as part of their compensation plans.

Many physician compensation formulas are designed to reward productivity. Obviously, the objective of rewarding productivity is to encourage physician production that results in more money coming into the group. Experience has generally shown that rewarding individual physicians directly for their personal efforts increases productivity. If you don't believe this, ask the hospitals that purchased physician practices over the last ten years and put the physicians on straight salary. Most noticed a significant drop in physician productivity. There are always exceptions to this premise, and we don't mean to imply that physicians are only motivated by money, but it helps. Compensation based on production seems to work best for physicians who work less than full time.[9] Be sure to include oversight and administrative duties based on a physician's time committed to these activities. You may want to consider compensating for these activities separately from those for patient care to avoid paying individuals for more than 100 percent of their available time.[10] As a side note, morale is sometimes the top factor in job satisfaction for physicians, not compensation.[11]

Also, remember to include all revenue from professional services rendered under contract which may not show up in the practice management system that is normally used to track services and ultimately RVUs. These services, often provided to hospitals or other entities, take many forms, but they usually fall under the general category of medical director responsibilities or something similar. Honoraria may be included as well, depending on the group's policy toward that type of revenue. If the services being reimbursed cannot be tracked at the procedure code level, RVUs can be derived by converting the revenue to RVUs using the average value of an RVU for the group. The point is, be sure to capture all the services and account for them in RVUs.

Productivity can be tracked and counted in many different ways. Some of these include patient visits, cases, gross charges and collections, although some organizations are seeing a shift away from measuring gross charges in performance-based compensation plans.[12] One methodology that has become more popular in recent years is the counting of RVUs as an indicator of physician productivity. Currently, the Medicare RBRVS system is the most common system and is useful in supporting a RVU productivity allocation system. As explained in other portions of this book, the RBRVS RVUs are broken down into three components (physician work, practice expense and malpractice) for each service provided. To reward individual physician productivity, it would make sense to use only that portion of the RVUs that relate to the physicians work. All of this assumes the practice has the capability to track the individual physician charges, break them down into work RVUs and then allocate them to the physician.

While not as common as using Medicare's RVU scale, some groups have decided to modify the Medicare scale or develop their own proprietary scale to provide incentives for certain behavior or to achieve objectives important to that group. One example is the Ohio Heart Health Center which developed its own RVU scale to deal with issues unique to its operations. By consensus, the group established a system of relative value units weighted by time to appropriately value each physician's work product. Its philosophy is that everyone's time is equally valuable; therefore the group ignores the other variables used to derive the work component of the RVU. In this group's system, the RVU for a new patient consult approximates that for a left heart catherization.[13]

Exhibit 5.1 demonstrates the difference in average Total RVUs versus Work RVUs for a few of the more common primary care

EXHIBIT 5.1. Difference Between Work and Average Total RVUs for Selected Specialties

Specialty	Average Total RVUs	Work RVUs	Work: Total Ratio
Family Practice w/o OB	8,095	3,963	0.49
Internal Medicine	7,061	3,917	0.55
Pediatrics	8,141	4,044	0.50
General Surgery	11,971	6,365	0.53
Orthopedics	14,995	7,229	0.48
OB/GYN	12,281	6,481	0.53

Source: MGMA Physician Compensation and Production Survey: 2001 Report Based on 2000 Data

and surgical specialties in MGMA's *Physician Compensation and Production Survey: 2001 Report Based on 2000 Data,* Tables 44 and 50. Once the RVUs by physician are determined, it is fairly easy to use them to allocate collections or profits.

Exhibit 5.2 demonstrates the totaling of a physician's procedures and the calculation of RVUs by procedure. This should be done for each physician and nonphysician provider included in the compensation plan.

Exhibit 5.3 shows the work RVUs by physician for a six-physician practice. The RVUs are then used to divide and allocate the practice's collections or profits, depending on how the compensation formula is structured.

A single-specialty primary care practice might not want to worry about allocation of expenses, and might assume that everyone is more or less equally responsible for expenses. This practice would then agree to divide the profits based on a pro rata share of the work RVUs. Column D in Exhibit 5.4 would support this calculation. This could be calculated monthly and rolled up with a quarterly or annual reconciliation.

Allocation of compensation or adding incentives by comparing physician RVUs against established benchmarks may be a way to provide incentives for certain behaviors. In the example in Exhibit 5.5, the practice wants to encourage physician productivity by rewarding performance above certain benchmarks. MGMA survey median work RVU data are used to establish the benchmarks in this example.

Don't forget that the pool of dollars available for distribution is generally finite. When you give some money to selected physicians as a reward, you have to take it from somewhere else. Practices that routinely distribute all profit as physician compensation will be "redistributing" compensation among the physicians under this benchmarking example. All of the physicians in the example exceeded the benchmark. Since the total available compensation didn't increase in this example, we merely shifted the existing money to the physicians who exceeded their benchmarks by the greatest margins, and then allocated their new "share" of the fixed pie of available dollars. You can imagine the

EXHIBIT 5.2. Calculation of RVUs for an Individual Physician's Procedures

Physician ID#

Specialty: Family Practice

CPT code	Description	Frequency	RVUs Per CPT Code					Frequency Adjusted RVU Totals			
			Work	Practice Expense	Mal-Practice	Totals		Work	Practice Expense	Mal-Practice	Totals
99202	Office, outpatient, new	243	0.88	0.77	0.05	1.70		214	187	12	413
99203	Office, outpatient, new	195	1.34	1.12	0.08	2.54		261	218	16	495
99204	Office, outpatient, new	107	2.00	1.51	0.10	3.61		214	162	11	386
99212	Office, outpatient, est.	707	0.45	0.53	0.02	1.00		318	375	14	707
99213	Office, outpatient, est.	1583	0.67	0.69	0.03	1.39		1061	1092	47	2200
99214	Office, outpatient, est.	424	1.10	1.04	0.04	2.18		466	441	17	924
99223	Initial hospital care	144	2.99	1.08	0.10	4.17		431	156	14	600
99232	Subsequent hosp	270	1.06	0.39	0.03	1.48		286	105	8	400
99233	Subsequent hosp	90	1.51	0.55	0.05	2.11		136	50	5	190
Other	Misc. Procedures	1725	0.45	0.53	0.02	1.00		776	914	35	1725
	Totals	5488						4163	3700	179	8041
	Average RVUs Per Code							0.76	0.67	0.03	1.47

EXHIBIT 5.3. RVUs by Physician for a Group Practice

	A	B	C	D	E	F
1						
2	**Physician**					
3		**Specialty**	**Total Work RVUs**	**% Total**	**Total RVUs**	**% Total**
4						
5	A	Family Practice w/o OB	3963	0.124	8095	0.129
6	B	Internal Medicine	3917	0.122	7061	0.113
7	C	Pediatrics	4044	0.126	8141	0.130
8	D	General Surgery	6365	0.199	11971	0.191
9	E	Orthopedics	7229	0.226	14995	0.240
10	F	OB/GYN	6481	0.203	12281	0.196
11						
12		**Totals**	31999		62544	

EXHIBIT 5.4. Allocation of Practice Net Revenue (Collections) by Work RVUs

	A	B	C	D
1				
2	Annual Practice Net Revenue =			$3,361,000
3				
4	**Physician**	**Specialty**	**% Work RVUs**	**Revenue Per Physician**
5				
6	A	Family Practice w/o OB	0.124	$416,252
7	B	Internal Medicine	0.122	$411,420
8	C	Pediatrics	0.126	$424,760
9	D	General Surgery	0.199	$668,545
10	E	Orthopedics	0.226	$759,295
11	F	OB/GYN	0.203	$680,729
12				
13			1.000	$3,361,000

EXHIBIT 5.5. Variation on the Profit Allocation Using RVU Benchmarks

	A	B	C	D	E	F	G
	Physician	**Specialty**	**Actual Work RVUs**		**MGMA Median RVUs Work**		**Actual/ Benchmark**
5	A	Family Practice w/o OB	3963		3834		1.034
6	B	Internal Medicine	3917		3790		1.034
7	C	Pediatrics	4044		3961		1.021
8	D	General Surgery	6365		6284		1.013
9	E	Orthopedics	7229		7014		1.031
10	F	OB/GYN	6481		6123		1.058
12	*In this example, everyone has exceeded the benchmark.*						

	A	B	C	D	E	F	G
	Physician	**Specialty**	**Profit/ Compensation Allocation**	**Actual/ Benchmark**	**Actual Salary**	**Collectable Cash Share %**	**Cash Distribution**
17	A	Family Practice w/o OB	$163,231	1.034	168,781	12.40%	$163,490
18	B	Internal Medicine	$161,336	1.034	166,821	12.26%	$161,592
19	C	Pediatrics	$166,567	1.021	170,065	12.50%	$164,734
20	D	General Surgery	$262,167	1.013	265,575	19.52%	$257,250
21	E	Orthopedics	$297,754	1.031	306,984	22.56%	$297,361
22	F	OB/GYN	$266,945	1.058	282,428	20.76%	$273,574
24	TOTALS:		$1,318,000		1,360,655	100.00%	$1,318,000

contribution a physician performing below the benchmark would have to make.

A group that wants to track productivity and has a comprehensive expense allocation system might use real or estimated collections per RVU to establish each physician's allocation of collected dollars in support of a cost allocation model. Column D in Exhibit 5.6 supports this calculation.

Using RVUs to Allocate Expenses

Some of the more comprehensive compensation models attempt to allocate expenses to physicians and/or departments within a practice. The simple equation is that expenses are deducted from allocated revenue, and the difference is the profit (compensation) for the physician. (It's never that simple, but readers will get the idea.)

There are at least two reasons for allocating expenses. One is a resource utilization issue; it ensures equity within a medical practice where physicians might be responsible for driving a greater or lesser share of expenses due to their specialties and/or volume. Another reason to allocate expenses is to encourage the judicious utilization of resources. A physician might think twice about requesting extra space, staff or equipment if required to pay the expense, and the expense isn't allocated (subsidized) across the group.

Exhibit 5.7 is a continuation of the example used earlier in Exhibit 5.4. It shows, by physician, the total of practice expense and malpractice RVUs and the allocation of all practice expenses in Column F.

An enhancement to this allocation of expenses is shown in Exhibit 5.8. This assumes the group wishes to allocate variable expenses by RVUs. These are the expenses that are more directly driven by productivity. The balance of the expense is allocated equally. This example assumes that 30 percent of the practice expenses are more or less directly related to production levels.

EXHIBIT 5.6. Allocation of Profit/Compensation by Work RVUs

	A	B	C	D
1				
2	Annual Practice Profit =		$1,318,000	
3				
4	**Physician**	**Specialty**	**% Work RVUs**	**Profit/ Compensation Allocation**
5				
6	A	Family Practice w/o OB	0.124	$163,231
7	B	Internal Medicine	0.122	$161,336
8	C	Pediatrics	0.126	$166,567
9	D	General Surgery	0.199	$262,167
10	E	Orthopedics	0.226	$297,754
11	F	OB/GYN	0.203	$266,945
12				
13			1.000	$1,318,000

EXHIBIT 5.7. Allocation of Practice Overhead (nonphysician) Expenses by RVUs

	A	B	C	D	E	F
1						
2	Practice Overhead Expenses		$2,043,000			
3						
4			**Practice Expense**			**Expense**
5	**Physician**	**Specialty**	**& Malpractice RVUs**			**Allocation**
6						
7	A	Family Practice w/o OB	4132	0.14		$276,369
8	B	Internal Medicine	3144	0.10		$210,286
9	C	Pediatrics	4097	0.13		$274,028
10	D	General Surgery	5606	0.18		$374,957
11	E	Orthopedics	7766	0.25		$519,428
12	F	OB/GYN	5800	0.19		$387,932
13						
14		Totals	30545	1.00		$2,043,000

EXHIBIT 5.8. Practice Expenses Allocated Equally and By RVUs

Practice Overhead Expenses		$2,043,000					

Physician	Specialty	Allocation 30% Overhead Equally	Practice Expense & Malpractice RVUs		Expense Allocation	Total Expense Allocation
A	Family Practice w/o OB	$102,150	4132	0.14	$193,458	$295,608
B	Internal Medicine	$102,150	3144	0.10	$147,200	$249,350
C	Pediatrics	$102,150	4097	0.13	$191,819	$293,969
D	General Surgery	$102,150	5606	0.18	$262,470	$364,620
E	Orthopedics	$102,150	7766	0.25	$363,600	$465,750
F	OB/GYN	$102,150	5800	0.19	$271,553	$373,703
Total		$612,900	30545	1.00	$1,430,100	$2,043,000

CONCLUSION

There is no end to the number and design of compensation models. The examples above can be used to craft a full production and expense allocation model based on RVUs. A group might decide to split part of the production equally among the physicians and part of the distribution based on RVUs. An example of this would be a group that has a lot of ancillary income, but doesn't want to reward anyone directly for referrals to the ancillary services. The ancillary services profit (or loss) could be split equally, and the balance allocated on RVU productivity.

Almost any compensation formula can be designed to promote and reward certain behaviors. For instance, five percent of the practice's profits could be taken out of the general compensation pool and then reallocated based on patient satisfaction survey scores. Some practices reward for service longevity or administrative and governance participation.

The MGMA surveys track RVUs in a variety of ways. One could use these data as a benchmarking resource in compensation formulas. An example would be to set a physician salary level based on MGMA specialty medians, and then adjust the salary up or down based on how the physician compares to the median work RVUs.

The allocation of work units and expense units can be further enhanced (or complicated, depending on how you look at it) by using the geographic adjustment indicators (GPCI factors). This is covered in more detail in chapter 1, and it is up to the group to decide how material these factors are to the compensation calculations.

Finally, a word of warning: No compensation system is perfect—these plans generally require constant review and adjustment. Also keep in mind that almost any complex system might be subject to "gaming," which occurs when the participants understand the system so well that they can adjust their behavior inappropriately to enhance their compensation. Examples of this would be to churn patients intentionally to drive up volume through excessive revisits, to upcode services that will be routinely downcoded by the payers, and to perform services that generate RVUs but won't be reimbursed.

The use of RVUs in a compensation formula can be a valuable and useful tool. Just keep in mind it is only one of many "tools" that can be used to fine-tune a generally complex and frequently contentious activity.

DISCUSSION
Compiling CPT Data

How do you approach the initial compilation of CPT data on a per code basis and make it reasonably easy to maintain and use?

"I maintain a current RVU table in Excel that consists principally of codes relevant to our practice. At the end of each month, I take a charge extract of all units of service booked as charges by doctor, by location. I use the table to lookup the relevant code and match it up with the RVUs using the VLOOKUP function in Excel. The whole process takes from about one-half hour up to one hour and that includes the downloading and formatting. I then have RVUs by location which can be used for cost analysis and physician compensation."

—Jim Bush
Chief Financial Officer
Eye Health Services, Inc.

"I have found the simplest way to compile and maintain RVU and CPT data is through a canned software package and a download from your practice management software. In case that option is not available, I would recommend a data extraction from your practice management software into a comma- or tab-delimited format that can be used by any spreadsheet or database program. Depending upon the practice management system and the volume within your practice, this may be the simplest solution. CMS provides the current year RBRVS data in a similar format. Your individual data can be cross-referenced and combined with the CPT data using functions within each program. For example, use VLOOKUP in Excel to match the RVU to each CPT code."

—Robert W. Ellis, CPA, CMPE
Chief Financial Officer
Charlotte Orthopedic Specialists

"Easy to maintain and use? RBRVS? Physician compensation? Are we serious? Actually, this can be done if we are willing to assume that a relatively small amount of information is indicative of what a physician is producing, and the practice management system can track physician productivity by CPT code and code frequency. The assumption, which usually works better with the primary care specialty, is that 75 percent or more of the physician's activity is concentrated in about 20 to 25 codes. This information base can be used to extrapolate a reasonable estimate of total productivity.

"Use your practice management system to list by CPT code and frequency all services rendered by the physician. Set up a spreadsheet listing the top codes and the frequency that these codes were performed during a time period. The total frequency of these codes should represent 75 percent or more of all codes. Depending on what you want to track, assign a RBRVS value (total, practice expense, physician effort, etc.) to each code and multiply the frequency by the RBRVS value. The sum of all these values for all CPT codes used should be a representative sample of total activity. Solve for estimated total RBRVS units by first determining the sample percentage of the total frequency (frequency of sample codes divided by frequency of all codes), and then dividing this percentage number into the total of sample relative value codes used. This should provide a reasonable estimate of total RVUs being tracked that can be used in a compensation formula when splitting the cash pie among physicians.

"As initially stated, this works well if the majority of total number of CPT codes is concentrated in a manageable sample size. If not, the model will still work. It just needs to be expanded until the sample population is large enough to provide a reasonable statistical confidence level."

—*Jeffrey B. Milburn*
Senior Vice President
Colorado Springs Health Partners, PC

REAL-LIFE EXAMPLES

Real-Life Example #1

The following is a real-life example from the University of Iowa Community Medical Services, Inc. (UICMS) using RVUs as a production incentive in a salary-based system. In this practice's physician compensation package, RVUs make up 10 percent of the physicians' base salaries, known as their "production incentive." A target is set—usually a standard one based on both MGMA's benchmarks from its survey reports and the 1996 Medicare RBRVS prior to the transitioning of RVUs by HCFA. In this case, the target was determined from the MGMA *Physician Compensation and Production Survey: 1998 Report Based on 1997 Data,* "Table 46, Physician Total RBRVS Units (TC/PE Excluded) for Family Practice (without OB)." A rounded estimate between the mean (5,980) and the median (5,785) was used.

Once a physician is past the initial two-year guaranteed salary, 10 percent of his/her salary is withheld. On a quarterly basis, the practice looks at the RVU production per physician. Physicians who are at or above target each receive the entire amount withheld for that quarter. Physicians who are below the target each lose 10 percent of the amount withheld for each one percent below the target. If they are 10 percent or more below their targets, they do not receive any of the amounts withheld, though they each can make the production up in the next quarter. Each quarter is calculated on a year-to-date basis to avoid any fluctuations in RVU production due to vacations or seasonal trends. If, at the end of the year, physicians are below the target, they each lose a portion of their production incentive based on the above formula. It does not carry over into the next year.

If the physicians (including those still in their initial two-year guarantee period) are above their targets at year end, they each receive a bonus for the number of RVUs they achieve beyond their targets. The bonus is calculated at 50 percent of the cash collection value per RVU of the practice. In other words, the administrator takes the total collections for the entire practice (factoring out non-RVU producing collections such as lab, immunizations, drugs and supplies) and divides by the total number of RVUs for all providers. This gives the administrator the cash collections per RVU. The physicians then receive 50 percent of this amount multiplied by the number of RVUs they attain above their targets.

Exhibits 5.9 and 5.10 show examples of the calculations that the administrator uses to show the physicians how the above production incentives and bonuses are calculated. Note that the net cash receipts figure shown in both examples is obtained from the UICMS billing system. The group is able to determine the cash collected during any given time period for each of its clinics. (This is done on a clinic basis, as some of the clinics are rural health clinics, and the year end settlement comes as a lump sum for the practice and not per provider.) The administrator then simply prorates these collections between production charges (those generating RVUs) and nonproduction charges (supplies, labs, immunizations and drugs). Also added is any other medical revenue that the physicians may have produced (medical director fees, medical examiner fees, etc.). The equation looks like this:

$$
\begin{array}{l}
\text{Cash collected during the contract year} \\
-\ \text{Portion applicable to nonproduction charges} \\
+\ \text{Other Revenue} \\
\hline
=\ \text{Net Collections for Bonus Calculation} \\[4pt]
\div\ \text{by Total RVUs for the practice during the} \\
\quad\text{same period} \\
\hline
=\ \text{Net Collections per RVU} \\[4pt]
\times\ 50\% \\
\hline
=\ \text{Bonus amount per RVU over the target}
\end{array}
$$

Physicians also receive RVUs for teaching and other outside income, which are worked into the above RVUs and used when comparing these providers' production to their targets.

Pros:

1. A portion of the physician's salary is based on production.

2. Bonus calculations take into account both the physician's production and the collections of the practice.

3. Physicians have an incentive to produce once they are at the 90 percent of target level.

Cons:

1. The bonus is not dependent on the bottom line of the practice.

2. Through no fault of the physicians, the patient population in rural towns may not be great enough for them to reach their targets. This makes the goals unattainable and reduces the incentive to increase practice size.

3. The percentage of salary at risk may not provide the necessary incentives for all physicians to attempt to meet or exceed the target.

4. The withholding and calculation of the 10 percent production incentive is confusing to many physicians.

According to Brian Roth, the group's comptroller:

"This model was developed when UICMS was first incorporated in 1996 and has remained our base model since. The group is currently considering looking at developing other models which will create win-win situations for both the practice and the physician. We need to develop a new model which will continue to attract quality physicians by providing them the opportunity to earn incentives while contributing to the financial well-being of the practice."

Real-Life Example #2

For Terry Brennan of Resource Management Associates, LLC, it was an easy decision for one of his client organizations to use the work component of the RVU (denoted WRVU) since it was established by independent parties and refined substantially to give the profession its best measurement tool to date.

EXHIBIT 5.9. Scenario #1—Target Exceeded

COMPENSATION PLAN EXAMPLE—PROFESSIONAL PRODUCTION ONLY

General Information:

Assumed Base Compensation:		$	145,000
Base Salary	80%	$	116,000
Productivity Incentive	10%	$	14,500
Quality Incentive	3%	$	4,350
Citizenship Incentive	2%	$	2,900
Group Management Incentive	5%	$	7,250
Total Compensation	100%	$	145,000
Professional Production Target:			5,900 RVUs
Net Cash Receipts for the Year:		$	250,000

In the scenario below, assume the Quality, Citizenship and Group Management incentives are being paid in full.

SCENARIO #1: Physician **exceeds** professional production target by 5% or 295 RVUs (i.e., produced 6,195 RVUs)

Base Salary	80%	$	116,000.00
Productivity Incentive			
Amount for meeting target	10%	$	14,500.00
Incentive for exceeding target		$	5,953.10 [1]
Quality Incentive	3%	$	4,350.00
Citizenship Incentive	2%	$	2,900.00
Group Management Incentive	5%	$	7,250.00
Total Compensation	100%	$	150,953.10

[1] Formula to Calculate Incentive Amount:

Total RVUs Produced		6,195
Production Target		5,900
RVUs Exceeding Target		295 RVUs
Net Cash Receipts	$	250,000
Divided by Total RVUs Produced		6,195
Net Cash Value per RVU	$	40.36
	×	50%
50% of Net Cash Value per RVU	$	20.18

Incentive for Exceeding Target:

RVUs Exceeding Target		295 RVUs
50% of Net Cash Value per RVU	$	20.18
Incentive for Exceeding Target	$	5,953.10

Note: When the professional production target is exceeded, the incentive calculation is based on both the RVUs produced and the net cash receipts of the clinic. In contrast, when the professional production target is not achieved, the production incentive is reduced based on the percentage amount that RVUs produced is below the target (production incentive is reduced 10% for each percentage point the RVUs produced is below the target).

EXHIBIT 5.10. Scenario #2—Target Not Achieved

COMPENSATION PLAN EXAMPLE—PROFESSIONAL PRODUCTION ONLY

General Information:

Assumed Base Compensation:		$	145,000
Base Salary	80%	$	116,000
Productivity Incentive	10%	$	14,500
Quality Incentive	3%	$	4,350
Citizenship Incentive	2%	$	2,900
Group Management Incentive	5%	$	7,250
Total Compensation	100%	$	145,000
Professional Production Target:			5,900 RVUs
Net Cash Receipts for the Year:		$	250,000

In the scenario below, assume the Quality, Citizenship and Group Management incentives are being paid in full.

SCENARIO #2: Physician **achieves only 95%** of professional production target (i.e., produced 5,605 RVUs)

Base Salary	80%	$ 116,000.00	
Productivity Incentive			
Amount if Target had			
been Achieved	10%	$ 14,500.00	
Deduction for not Achieving Target		$ (7,250.00) [2]	
Quality Incentive	3%	$ 4,350.00	
Citizenship Incentive	2%	$ 2,900.00	
Group Management Incentive	5%	$ 7,250.00	
Total Compensation	100%	$ 137,750.00	

[2] **Formula to Calculate Deduction from Incentive:**

Percentage Points Below Target:

Production Achieved	95%
Target	100%
Percentage Points Below Target	-5%

Percentage to Reduce Productivity Incentive:

Percentage Points Below Target	-5%
Reduction of Productivity Incentive	
per Percentage Points below Target ×	10%
Percentage to Reduce Productivity Incentive	-50%

Dollar Amount to Reduce Productivity Incentive:

Original Productivity Incentive	
(10% of Base Comp)	$14,500.00
Percentage to Reduce Productivity Incentive	-50%
Dollar Amount to Reduce Productivity Incentive	$(7,250.00)

Note: When the professional production target is exceeded, the incentive calculation is based on both the RVUs produced and the net cash receipts of the clinic. In contrast, when the professional production target is not achieved, the production incentive is reduced based on the percentage amount that RVUs produced is below the target (production incentive is reduced 10% for each percentage point the RVUs produced is below the target).

According to Brennan:

"The actual development process spanned some 18 months and countless iterations to arrive at a product that would sustain a consensus. We are now at a point, as with most plans, where some changes need to be made. These changes basically reflect what would be done differently if we were just beginning the process today.

"First, due to significant differences in productivity, the amount of money distributed equally should be limited to that which is a function of the group rather than the individual; specifically, the technical component profit is the only thing that should be shared equally by the partners. Everything else should be based on individual productivity. Employed physicians do not have access to the technical component profit bonus pool now, nor would they in the revised edition.

"Second, the amount of money necessary to buy out of call should be increased to the point where it is almost prohibitively expensive since this is by far the most difficult work. In fact, I would recommend that if someone wants to give up call, they should resign their partner/shareholder status and be treated as an employed physician at a substantially reduced rate of compensation and limited access to the professional fee bonus pools.

"Finally, I would recommend that as many costs as possible be tracked by individual physician and treated as a direct cost, as opposed to being allocated as overhead. This is, without a doubt, the most effective way to reduce unnecessary expenditures and increase physician satisfaction, since they can manage their expenses better than anyone else and at the same time get what they want for the money."

This particular compensation plan, as follows, has specific goals and objectives that clearly spell out the expectations and rules of the game.

Compensation Plan

Purpose: The compensation plan encompasses benefits as well as cash distributed in an equitable manner that recognizes individual contributions and preferences in a group practice while fostering collaboration, growth and a level of quality which sets the group apart from the competition.

Goals	Objectives
Be simple to understand and monitor	• Measure well defined variables: revenue, expense, WRVUs, meeting/drive times
Encourage revenue maximization	• Heavily weighted toward productivity; no cap on compensation • Annual compensation fluctuates based on productivity by individual
Encourage minimal resource consumption	• Account for resource consumption by individual (CME, car, cell phone) where feasible; distribute remaining overhead in proportion to the percentage of WRVUs generated by each physician
Be equitable regardless of subspecialty and payer mix	• Utilize only the work component of RVUs to measure productivity • Distribute revenue based on WRVUs • Create bonus pools by subspecialty • Share technical component revenue in excess of expense, proportionately amongst shareholders based on percentage of WRVUs to total shareholder WRVUs
Be equitable regardless of location	• Ensure equal access to patients, internal and external referrals, staff and facilities
Recognize administrative contributions to the group	• Compensate physicians based on time spent using average WRVUs/hour across all physicians

Recognize lifestyle choices	• Physicians can influence income via productivity • Individuals can buy out of call at predetermined rates • Physicians can control expenses at their discretion whenever feasible (CME, car, cell phone) • Employee contract for non-shareholders provides access to bonus pools on a reduced basis with no cap on earnings
Encourage outreach activities	• Compensate for drive time and development time (availability) using average WRVUs/hour across all physicians

Furthermore, based on the goals and objectives previously agreed upon, the following principles are used to determine compensation under the plan.

- A standard base salary for all physicians will be set at a level which represents approximately 50 percent to 60 percent of total cash compensation with incentive bonus payments comprising approximately 40 percent to 50 percent of total cash compensation.
- Base salary for shareholders for the first year will be set at the current salary for shareholders or the standard base salary which ever is higher, and adjusted down if necessary in the second year of the plan. Amounts in excess of the standard base salary will be considered advances on the bonus and may continue for the first year or as long as the bonus equals or exceeds the amount of the advance.
- Physician employees (nonshareholders) will receive the same standard base salary as shareholders. Physician employees will be eligible to receive 25 percent of the bonus they would have received if they were shareholders, except that physician employees will not share in any revenue from technical component services.
- In addition to base salary, noncash compensation expenses will be tracked by the physician for the purpose of determining total compensation. These expenses include pension contributions, profit sharing contributions, health insurance, dental insurance, vision

insurance, life insurance, group disability insurance and other non-cash compensation expenses as approved by the board. These items will be excluded from a physician's direct expenses.

- Automobile, CME in excess of $7,500 per year, cellular phone expense and other expenses as approved by the board that can be tracked to a specific physician will be referred to as physician direct expenses and will reduce eligible bonus amounts dollar for dollar prior to distribution to that physician from the bonus pool(s). CME monies that are unspent at the end of the fiscal year will be forfeited.

- The work component of the RVUs (WRVUs) will be used to determine each physician's proportionate share of the respective bonus pools. Professional services rendered under contract to hospitals or other entities and funds received for services to hospitals or other entities (such as medical directorships) referred to as Management Contract Revenue will be converted to WRVUs for purposes of determining that physician's share of the bonus pool. Travel time (and time available, if appropriate) to outreach locations, time spent in meetings (such as corporation, executive committee and others) as well as any other activities as may be determined by the board will be converted to WRVUs. WRVUs will neither be given to the president for corporation meetings nor to the executive committee for executive committee meetings since these individuals receive cash in lieu of WRVUs for those activities. The conversion will be calculated by first obtaining the average WRVUs for a physician for a one-year period including shareholder and physicians employees. The average physician WRVUs per year will then be divided by an average number of hours worked for the time period (for example, 2,668 hours: 46 weeks × 58 hours/week allowing six weeks for time off and CME).

- Professional fee revenue will be allocated to each physician in proportion to the WRVUs generated by each physician as a percentage of the total WRVUs of the group directly attributable to those professional fees.

- Group overhead expenses such as rent, the business office, shared personnel and similar expenses not directly attributable to any physician will be allocated to each physician in proportion to the WRVUs generated by each physician as a percentage of the total WRVUs for the group.

- The total amount available for distribution will be determined by subtracting total physician expenses from total physician revenue and then adding technical component profit.

- The total amount available for distribution will then be divided into the following bonus pools:
  —Administration (president/executive committee)
  —Technical component
  —Professional

Administration Pool

The president of the corporation will receive $10,000 per year in addition to his/her share of the other bonus pools in recognition of time spent on corporation activities in lieu of receiving an equivalent amount of WRVUs. Likewise, the executive committee including the president and the past-president will receive $10,000 per year in addition to their shares of the other bonus pools in recognition of time spent on corporation activities in lieu of receiving an equivalent amount of WRVUs.

Technical Component Pool

Every shareholder physician will share in the profit from technical component services based on his percentage of total WRVUs to the total WRVUs of the shareholder group (profit being defined as technical component revenue minus technical component expense).

Professional Pool

The professional fee bonus pools will be determined by subtracting the technical component and president/executive committee pools from the total amount available for distribution. The remaining pools will be allocated proportionate amounts based on the number of WRVUs in each pool as a percentage of the total WRVUs. Likewise, each physician will receive a proportionate share of the respective pools based on his/her WRVUs in that pool as a percentage of the total WRVUs in that pool.

The amount actually distributed to each physician will be determined by the following formula:

[Percentage of professional fee pools + percentage of technical component pool + administrative pool] –

[advances toward bonus + physician direct expense]

= remainder for distribution

Bonuses will be determined once a year, at the end of the fiscal year. Interim bonus calculations performed prior to fiscal year end will be considered estimates, and each interim calculation will be done on a cumulative basis—the intent being to bonus based on the experience of an entire year. Accordingly, interim bonus payments will be considered advances on the final year end bonus.

The following policy only pertains to employed physicians who have become partners in the Group Practice, and provides an option for them to reduce their participation in call on weekends as follows:

- **Age 50–54:** Call for weekends may be reduced by one-third. The individual assigning call will compute the number of normal call requirements over a year in relation to the number of physicians currently employed. The physician desiring to reduce his/her call would then decide if the reduction would occur during one time period or would be spread across a year. Assignment of call would be distributed among all other physicians participating in call. This would not pertain to weekday call. *Selection of this option would result in a reduction in base salary of $4,000.*

- **Age 55–60:** Call for weekends may be reduced by one-half of the normal call schedule (the call schedule prior to any reductions under this plan). The individual assigning call will compute the number of normal call requirements over a year in relation to the number of physicians currently employed. The physician desiring to reduce his/her call must decide if the reduction would occur during one time period or would be spread across a year. Assignment of call would be distributed among all other physicians participating in call. This option would not pertain to weekday call. *Selection of this option would result in an additional reduction in base salary of $4,000 or a total of $8,000 if the individual had not previously exercised an option to reduce call under this plan.*

- **Age 60+ and/or completion of 20 years of employment:** Weekend call may be suspended for physicians 60 or more years of age or who have worked within the practice as a partner for 20 years. This option does not affect weekday call requirements. *Selection of this option will result in an additional reduction in base salary of $8,000 or a total of $16,000 if the individual had not previously exercised an option to reduce call under this plan.*

So, what is the methodology behind this carefully designed compensation plan? It looks like this:

1. Derive actual work relative value units (WRVUs) for each physician by multiplying procedure frequency (from the practice management system analysis of services report) by Medicare WRVUs (from CMS Web site for year in question), then add WRVUs per physician to obtain total WRVUs from professional services.

2. Derive dollar value per WRVU by dividing cash receipts (from practice management system and accounting system net of technical component revenue, hospital director, hospital payments, revenues etc.) by total WRVUs from #1.

3. Convert hospital payments to hospital WRVUs using information from #2.

4. Add actual WRVUs to hospital WRVUs to obtain total WRVUs.

5. Derive percentage of total WRVUs for each physician from #4.

6. Derive average WRVUs per hour by dividing total WRVUs by hours based on 2,668 hours per year (58 hours/week × 46 weeks).

7. Derive meeting and drive/availability time WRVUs by multiplying average WRVUs per hour by total hours for each category.

8. Derive technical component profit by subtracting technical component expenses (from accounting system) from technical component revenue (from practice management system).

9. Multiply net professional revenue by physician from #2 by percentage of actual WRVUs obtained in #1 and then add hospital revenue to obtain distributed revenue by physician.

10. Subtract standard base salary from actual salary (and bonus paid if applicable) to obtain advance toward bonus amount.

11. Subtract physician actual salaries, bonuses, (if applicable) and direct expenses, as well as technical component expense

and other miscellaneous items as necessary from total expenses to obtain overhead amount to be shared; then multiply this amount by each physician's percentage of WRVUs obtained in #5 (excluding meeting and drive time WRVUs) to obtain shared overhead amount by physician.

12. Add physician standard base salary, benefits and shared overhead to obtain total physician expense; then subtract total physician expense from total distributed revenue by physician from #9 to obtain amount available for distribution (surplus).

13. Segregate WRVUs from #4 and #7 above into subspecialty professional fee pools. Then determine each physician's percentage of the respective pools and each pool's percentage of total WRVUs.

14. Subtract technical component profit and president/executive committee payments from #8. Then multiply remainder by percentage amounts from #13 to obtain amount available for distribution by pool.

15. Multiply each physician's percentage of the respective pools from #13 by amount available for distribution from each of the respective pools from #14 to obtain each physician's share.

16. Segregate WRVUs from #13 into shareholder and non-shareholder groups; calculate each shareholder's percentage of the total WRVUs for the shareholder group.

17. Multiply the technical component profit from #8 by each physician's shareholder percentage from #16 to obtain each shareholder's share of technical component profit.

18. Add each physician's share of the respective bonus pools from #15 to each shareholder's share of technical component profit and president/executive committee payments to obtain bonus amount due by physician.

19. From #18, subtract physician direct expenses and advances toward bonus by physician to derive remainder for distribution by physician.

Other Resources

Physician's Compensation: Measurement, Benchmarking and Implementation by Lucy R. Carter and Sara S. Lankford. John Wiley & Sons 2000.

Physician Compensation Arrangements: Management & Legal Trends by Dan Zismer and Daniel K. Zismer. Aspen Publishers 1999.

Physician Compensation: Models for Aligning Financial Goals and Incentives, 2nd edition by Kenneth Hekman. Englewood, CO: Medical Group Management Association (MGMA) 2002.

Notes

1. Cejka, S., Coleman, LK. (1997). Don't Get Decapitated by a Poor Physician Compensation Plan. Today's Internist, 38(2):12–8.

2. Alper, M. (2001, September). Risking It All: Successful Compensation Strategies for Provider Organizations. Group Practice Journal, 50(9): 20–4.

3. Redling, B. (1999, November). Physician Compensation Plans: Small Groups are Different. Medical Group Management Update, 38(21): 10.

4. Nelson, JL., Rider, CT., Biermann, JE., Schwartz, SD. (2001, September). Physician Compensation Models in Large Medical Groups. Group Practice Journal, 50(8): 16–9.

5. Gammel, JD. (1996, September/October). How to Evaluate the Value of Production-Based Compensation Programs. Group Practice Journal, 45(5):22, 24–6.

6. (2001, April). Measuring Physician Production: Ways to Calculate the Top Line. Financial Management Strategies for Medical Offices, pp 3–4.

7. (2001, April). Measuring Physician Production: Ways to Calculate the Top Line. Financial Management Strategies for Medical Offices, pp 3–4.

8. Jacob, JA. (2001, August). Modest Compensation Gains for Most Doctors. American Medical News, 44(30):25

9. Nelson, JL., Rider, CT., Biermann, JE., Schwartz, SD. (2001, September). Physician Compensation Models in Large Medical Groups. Group Practice Journal, 50(9): 16–9.

10. Cejka, S., Coleman, LK. (1997, March/April). Don't Get Decapitated by a Poor Physician Compensation Plan. Today's Internist, 38(2):12–8.

11. Versal, N. (2001, August). It Pays To Produce. Modern Physician 5(11):21–4.

12. Versal, N. (2001, August). It Pays To Produce. Modern Physician, 5(11):21–4.

13. Kereiakes, DJ, (1999, January/February). Into the Third Millennium: The Changing Face of Cardiology Practice. The Journal of Cardiovascular Management, 10(1):20–23.

Glossary

ADA (American Dental Association)
The American Dental Association (ADA) is the professional association of dentists committed to the public's oral health, ethics, science and professional advancement; leading a unified profession through initiatives in advocacy, education, research and the development of standards. Learn more about the ADA by visiting its website at www.ada.org.

AMA (American Medical Association)
The American Medical Association (AMA) is an association for physicians and is the nation's leader in promoting professionalism in medicine and setting standards for medical education, practice and ethics. Learn more about the AMA by visiting its website at www.ama-assn.org.

ASA (American Society of Anesthesiologists)
The American Society of Anesthesiologists (ASA) is an educational, research and scientific association of physicians organized to raise and maintain the standards of the medical practice of anesthesiology and improve the care of the patient. Founded in 1905, ASA is the foremost advocate for all patients who require anesthesia for relief from pain. Learn more about the ASA by visiting its website at www.asahq.org.

Adjusted Charges
Adjusted charges are the total amounts expected to be paid by patients or third-party payers. This figure can be calculated by taking gross charges and subtracting the adjustments from third-party payers and charge restrictions from Medicare/Medicaid.

Benchmark

A benchmark is the ongoing process of establishing a standard of excellence and comparing activities to that standard, whether it is internal or external to the organization.

Capitation Contract

Capitation contracts are a type of third-party payer contract that, in theory, are focused on preventive services and health maintenance. Capitated contracts are concerned with utilization of services and assumption for risk of providing patient care under a predetermined payment arrangement. The payer offers to pay a practice a predetermined amount per covered plan member per month, and in return the practice assumes most or all of the risk associated with those patients' care. The practice receives those funds regardless of whether the member visits the clinic or utilizes any services. Capitated contracts, which always contain an element of risk, include HMO, Medicare and Medicaid capitation contracts.

CDT (*Current Dental Terminology*)

Current Dental Terminology (CDT) codes are alphanumeric labels assigned to dental procedures for the purpose of billing and documentation. CDT codes are to dental procedures what CPT codes are to medical procedures.

CFTE (*Clinical Full-Time Equivalent*)

A clinical FTE (CFTE) provider is defined by the minimum number of *clinical* hours the practice considers to be the minimum for a normal *clinical* workweek. *Clinical work* includes time the provider devotes to patient care and supporting activities, such as medical records update, consultation with other providers, preparation for clinical and/or surgical procedures, patient phone contact, etc.

CMS (*Centers for Medicare and Medicaid Services*)

The Centers for Medicare and Medicaid Services (CMS) is a federal agency within the U.S. Department of Health and Human Services. CMS runs the Medicare and Medicaid programs—two national health care programs that benefit about 75 million Americans. Together with the Health Resources and Services

Administration, CMS also runs the State Children's Health Insurance Program (SCHIP), a program that is expected to cover many of the approximately 10 million uninsured children in the United States. CMS was formerly known as the Health Care Financing Administration (HCFA).

Code Ranges

A code range is a group of codes that encompass related procedures or services. Examples of ranges include surgery codes 10040 to 69990, evaluation and management (E&M) codes 99201 to 99499, and medicine codes 90281 to 99199. The logic behind this basic categorization is that charges and RVUs tend to be similar within the same range of codes. Naturally the code ranges would have to be much smaller than these broad categories in order for this logic to bear itself out.

Conversion Factor

A conversion factor is simply the dollar amount paid per RVU by third-party payers. It converts RVUs into money for reimbursement of medical procedures.

Cost-Based Fee Schedule

A cost-based fee schedule is one that reflects the actual cost the practice incurs to provide the service or procedure to the patient. Determine the cost for each procedure and add a percentage to it to act as a buffer against discounts and bad debts. The "cost-plus" amount now becomes the practice's standard fee for that procedure.

CPR (*Customary, prevailing and reasonable*)

Customary, prevailing and reasonable (CPR) charges were the traditional fee-for-service rates and the universally accepted method of reimbursement until the advent of managed care and of the RBRVS and RVUs.

CPT (Common Procedural Terminology) codes

CPT codes are five-digit numerical codes used to indicate the types of services and procedures performed by a medical care provider. Currently published in the 4th edition of *Common Procedure*

Terminology, CPT codes are copyrighted by the American Medical Association.

Discounted Fee-For-Service

The discounted FFS is one of the simpler third-party payer contracts because it is really just a percentage off the practice's own charges. Contractors might offer percentage rates or reimbursement for procedures and services that are a discount off the medical practice's usual fee schedule. The contract might pay, for example, 80 percent of the group's current fee schedule; or, as a twist, the contract would pay the lesser of the group's fee or the contracted rate.

Encounter

An encounter is a documented, face-to-face contact between a patient and a provider who exercises independent judgement in the provision of services to an individual. If the patient with the same diagnosis sees two different providers on the same day, it is one encounter. If a patient sees two different providers on the same day for two different diagnoses, then it is considered two encounters.

Factor of the RBRVS

A factor of the RBRVS is a type of third-party payer contract that uses a percentage of the RBRVS or a (conversion) factor of Medicare, meaning that the rates are above or below Medicare's rates by some set amount. For example, a contract may be 140 percent (the factor is 1.40) or 85 percent (a factor of 0.85) of Medicare's standard reimbursement.

Fee-for-Service

Gross charges at the practice's established undiscounted rates.

Fee Schedule

A fee schedule is a list of the practice's standard rates for providing procedures and services to patients. The three main types of fee schedules are historical-based, market-based and cost-based.

FTE (Full-Time Equivalent)

According to MGMA, a full-time equivalent (FTE) physician or nonphysician provider works whatever number of hours the practice considers to be the minimum for a normal workweek, which could be 37.5, 40, 50 hours or some other standard.

GPCIs (Geographic Practice Cost Indices)

Geographic Practice Cost Indices (GPCIs) are adjustment factors created by CMS to account for the geographic cost difference across the United States. These factors are used to calculate Medicare reimbursements when multiplied by the RVUs associated with each CPT code. GPCIs are divided into the same three components as the RVUs within the RBRVS: physician work, practice expense and malpractice.

Gross Charges

Gross patient charges are the full dollar value, at the practice's established undiscounted rates, of services provided to all patients before reduction by charitable adjustments, professional courtesy adjustments, contractual adjustments, employee discounts, bad debts, etc. For both Medicare participating and nonparticipating providers, gross charges should include the practice's full undiscounted charge and not the Medicare limiting charge.

HCFA (Health Care Financing Administration)

HCFA changed its name to CMS in 2001. See CMS for further information.

HCPCS (HCFA's Common Procedure Coding System)

HCFA's Common Procedure Coding System (HCPCS) is a standardized method or system for reporting professional services, procedures and supplies. HCPCS codes are typically paid on a flat rate and therefore do not have RVUs assigned to the codes, since none are required to calculate a reimbursement rate. Even though HCFA changed its name to CMS in 2001, as of this writing, HCPCS has not yet followed suit.

HMO (*Health Maintenance Organization*)

Health maintenance organizations (HMOs) are typically health plans that utilize primary care physicians as gatekeepers, but HMOs can also be health plans that place some or most of the risk of patient care expenses onto the providers. In other words, an HMO is an insurance company that accepts responsibility for providing and delivering a predetermined set of comprehensive health maintenance and treatment services to a voluntarily enrolled population for a negotiated and fixed periodic premium.

Key Indicators

Key indicators, as used in this publication, are the calculations used to determine and compare physician productivity and cost effectiveness. These calculations are usually determined on a per unit basis, which allows for a more equitable comparison than totals, because it allows data to be viewed on a level playing field. The following is a list and description of the key indicators used in this book. This list is by no means exhaustive, but is added here as a starting point for analyzing data. Unless otherwise noted, all of these calculations can be done at the group, specialty and/or provider levels by using only the data associated with the selected level of detail.

Charge/FTE

The charge/FTE is the average charge per FTE provider, calculated by dividing the total charges by the total FTE count.

$$\frac{\text{Total Charges}}{\text{Total FTE count}}$$

Charge/patient

The charge/patient is the average charge produced per patient visit. It is calculated by dividing the total gross charges by the number of patients seen.

$$\frac{\text{Total Charges}}{\text{Number of Patients}}$$

Charge/procedure

The charge/procedure is the average charge produced per procedure for the clinic. It is calculated by dividing the clinic's total gross charges by the number of procedures completed to produce the gross charges

$$\frac{\text{Total Charges}}{\text{Number of Procedures}}$$

Charge/RVU

The charge/RVU is the average charge per RVU and is calculated by dividing the total charges by the total RVUs. This allows the clinic to understand what they are charging for their services. If differences occur between specialties, this may indicate that the internal fee schedule needs to be reviewed.

$$\frac{\text{Total Charges}}{\text{Total RVUs Produced}}$$

Cost/Procedure

Based on a practice's Cost/RVU, the Cost/Procedure is the average cost for the clinic to provide a procedure or service. It can be compared with the reimbursement from a third-party payer to determine whether a contract will cover the cost to the clinic. It can be calculated using either the blended cost per RVU or the component cost per RVU.

$$RVU_{total} * Cost/RVU_{blended} = Cost/Procedure$$

or

$$(RVU_w * Cost/RVU_w) + (RVU_{pe} * Cost/RVU_{pe})$$
$$+ (RVU_m * Cost/RVU_m) = Cost/Procedure$$

Cost/RVU$_{blended}$

The blended Cost/RVU is the average cost per RVU. It is calculated by dividing the sum (Σ) of the practice's total expenses by the sum of the total RVUs produced within that practice during the same time period. This is an indication of the cost control vs. volume with a group or practice.

$$\frac{\Sigma \text{ Total expenses}}{\Sigma \text{ Total RVUs}}$$

Cost/RVU$_m$

The cost per malpractice RVU is calculated by dividing the sum of the total malpractice premium expense by the total malpractice RVUs. This indicates the cost of malpractice coverage per RVU.

$$\frac{\Sigma \text{ Total malpractice expenses}}{\Sigma \text{ Total RVU}_m}$$

Cost/RVU$_{pe}$

The cost per practice expense RVU is calculated by dividing the sum of total practice expenses by the sum of the total practice expense RVUs. This should be monitored as an indicator for cost vs. volume.

$$\frac{\Sigma \text{ Total practice expenses}}{\Sigma \text{ Total RVU}_{pe}}$$

Cost/RVU$_w$

The cost per work RVU is calculated by dividing the sum of the total provider compensation by the sum of the total work RVUs. This is an indication of what a practice is, on average, paying their providers per work RVU.

$$\frac{\Sigma \text{ Total provider compensation expenses}}{\Sigma \text{ Total RVU}_w}$$

Procedures/FTE

The procedures/FTE indicator is the average number of procedures billed per FTE provider. It is calculated by dividing the total procedures by the total FTE count.

$$\frac{\text{Total Procedures}}{\text{Total FTE count}}$$

Procedures/Patient

The procedures/patient indicator is the average number of procedures or services provided to each patient. It is calculated by dividing the total number of procedures by the number of patients seen during the same time period. This can give a clinic an idea of its patient mix complexity.

$$\frac{\text{Total Procedures}}{\text{Number of Patients}}$$

RVUs/FTE

The RVUs/FTE indicator is the average number of RVUs produced per FTE provider during a specific time period. It is calculated by dividing the total number of RVUs produced by the total FTE count. This indicator can be a good productivity measure by which to compare providers within a specialty.

$$\frac{\text{Total Charges}}{\text{Total FTE count}}$$

RVUs/Patient

RVUs/patient is the average number of RVUs produced per patient seen. It is calculated by dividing the total number of RVUs produced by the total number of patients seen. This can be a good indicator for patient mix complexity and may lead to the discovery of coding issues within the clinic if the result is higher than set standards.

$$\frac{\text{Total RVUs Produced}}{\text{Total Patients}}$$

RVUs/Procedure

The RVUs/procedure indicator is the average amount of RVUs produced during each procedure. It is calculated by dividing the total number of RVUs produced by the number of procedures completed. This can be a good indicator for both procedure and patient complexity.

$$\frac{\text{Total RVUs Produced}}{\text{Total Procedures}}$$

Managed Care Fee Schedule

A managed care fee schedule is a predetermined fee schedule for specific services offered to the practice by a third-party payer.

MCOs (*Managed Care Organizations*)
"Managed care organizations" (MCOs) is a generic phrase or term for managed care health plans, which include HMOs and PPOs (preferred provider organizations).

MGMA (*Medical Group Management Association*)
The Medical Group Management Association, founded in 1926, is the leading organization for professionals in medical practice management. Learn more about MGMA by visiting its website at www.mgma.com.

Modifiers
Modifiers are used, among other things, to adjust the reimbursement of a service or procedure to account for assistant surgeons, multiple procedures, bilateral procedures, etc. If the reimbursement is adjusted for a CPT code, it would be logical that the charge and associated RVUs would be similarly affected. Most medical procedure modifiers (with the primary exception of anesthesia codes) make adjustments by percentages rather than amounts.

Nonphysician Providers
Also referred to as midlevel providers, these are specially trained and licensed individuals, employed or contracted, who can provide medical care and billable services. Examples of nonphysician providers include the following:

- Audiologist;
- Certified Registered Nurse Anesthetist;
- Dietician/nutritionist;
- Midwife;
- Nurse practitioner;
- Occupational therapist;
- Optometrists;
- Perfusionist (surgical);
- Physical therapist;

- Physician assistant (primary care, nonsurgical or surgical);
- Psychologist;
- Social worker;
- Speech therapist; and
- Surgeon's assistant.

Physician

Any doctor of medicine (MD) or doctor of osteopathy (DO) who is duly licensed and qualified under the law of jurisdiction in which treatment is received.

Reimbursement

Reimbursement is compensation for procedures or services performed by the medical practice to a patient.

RBRVS (*Resource-Based Relative Value Scale*)

CMS's Resource-Based Relative Value Scale (RBRVS) includes all the CPT-4 codes, a brief description of each code and the RVUs associated with each code. It also contains CMS's common procedure coding system (HCPCS).

RTCU (*Relative Time-Cost Unit*)

The Relative Time-Cost Unit (RTCU) is a system similar to the RBRVS used for the valuation of dental procedures and the development of dental fees based on the provider effort initiated. This system incorporates personal cost, task mixes and task time into relative weights for valuation of dental procedures.

RUC (*RBRVS Update Committee*)

The RBRVS Update Committee is a standing committee that meets on a regular basis to discuss potential changes to the RVUs contained within the RBRVS.

RVPs (*Relative Values for Physicians*)

The St. Anthony/McGraw-Hill scale is called the Relative Values for Physicians (RVP). St. Anthony's *Complete RBRVS* publication provides values both for services that are contained in the

Medicare Physicians' Fee Schedule (MPFS) and for procedures and services that are either not yet reimbursable by Medicare or that are reimbursed on a flat fee basis, such as laboratory tests. The methodology used to develop the McGraw-Hill scale consisted of a random sample of physicians from across the United States who were asked to rate specific procedures as to time, skill, risk to the patient, risk to the provider and severity of illness of each. The main differences between the RVP scale and the RBRVS are that the RVP scale (a) does not break out the physician work component, (b) is a compilation of five independent scales (medicine, surgery, radiology/pathology, laboratory, and E&M) instead of one, and (c) is focused more on specialty care than primary care.

RVUs (*Relative Value Units*)

Relative value units (RVUs) are nonmonetary, relative units of measure that indicate the value of health care services and relative difference in resources consumed when providing different procedures and services. RVUs assign *relative* values or weights to medical procedures primarily for the purpose of reimbursement of services performed. They are used as a standardized method of analyzing resources involved in the provision of services or procedures.

RVU_m

RVU_m is the malpractice component of the total RVU. This component measures the risk involved in providing a service.

RVU_{pe}

RVU_{pe} is the practice expense component of the total RVU. This component measures the amount of resources attributed to overhead required to provide the service. This includes, but is not limited to, ancillary staff's time and effort and use of supplies and equipment.

RVU_w

RVU_w is the physician work component of the total RVU. This component is designed to measure a provider's skill and effort and the degree of decision-making complexity required for performing a procedure.

TCG (*Technical Consulting Groups*)

Technical consulting groups (TCGs) comprising more than 200 physicians were organized into 33 specialty-specific consulting groups to provide guidance on the study structure and to define physician work for the RBRVS and its RVUs.